The ABCs

How to Always Be Curly and Love It!

Curls of Wisdom from…

ADINA SHERMAN

Founder of Curly Girls Studio

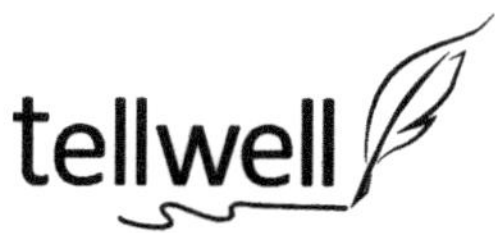

Tellwell Talent
www.tellwell.ca

ISBN
978-1-77302-332-8 (Hardcover)
978-1-77302-331-1 (Paperback)
978-1-77302-333-5 (eBook)

Table of Contents

Changing the way you look at your hair... one curl at a time.

— Curly Stylist Adina

Dedicated and a special thanks to:

All the curly girls and guys near and far with whom I have been fortunate enough to cross curly paths. I may have taught you, but from behind the chair I have also learned from your hair stories and experiences. You have helped me grow and inspired me to create a little take-home pamphlet, a project that has since grown into this book instead.

My very special and loyal regulars, from wavy to kinky curly, you light up my studio with your presence, life stories and laughter. I truly have the most amazing clients and best job in the world!

Deep appreciation and gratitude go to my very talented editors who are also curly girls. My starter, Deanna Dority, always "put in a good word for me," and my closer, Julie Caspersen, provided inspiration for the cover, did a final sweep of the text and helped me make it to the last page. I could not have done this without either of you.

A special thank you to Mrs. Armstrong. Your patience, guidance and professionalism as an educator is a true inspiration. I value every moment I had the privilege of being a student in your class.

I also dedicate this book to my creative spaces: Varadero – Barcelo Arenas Blancas, Be Live Los Morlas & Quatro Palmas; my locals: The Miller, The Keg and, of course, Starbucks; and the most peaceful places to be creative: Nicolston Dam and Via Rail.

The first shall be last and the last shall be first. A very special thank you and love go to my wonderful family who have stood by me through thick and thin without fail. I'm so very blessed to have you. Josh and Rachel, you give meaning to my life. I love you all more than words can say.

Intro

Welcome to Curly Girls Studio. Your coaching session is about to begin! My name is Adina, and *The ABCs: How to Always Be Curly and Love It!* is a guide written to help you do just that—learn to "Always Be Curly" and love it!

Any hair pattern that isn't straight, I consider a curl. I will refer to you, the reader, as a **curly** (or **curlies**) throughout the book. This book is for you if you have slightly wavy, wavy, curly or extremely curly hair. (Secret: A lot of what's in *The ABCs* can benefit a friend with straight hair, too. So do share!) Maybe you're in curly "hair despair" from any one of the following or a combination thereof:

- Heat damage from curling irons, flat irons, blow-dries or hot combs
- Chemical damage from relaxers or perms, or straightening systems
- Frizz, and can't control it
- Damage from color or highlights with "straightened ends" syndrome
- Struggle with multi-curl patterns
- Change in curl pattern from previous years
- Can't get good next-day curl
- Have great curls the first few hours when freshly washed and styled, then the curls drop and flop as the day goes on

Or maybe you're a curly who's confused about how to use styling products or just needs inspiration to bring out the best in your curls, whether they're big or small, zigzag or wavy. Or maybe you're a parent challenged with a curly child.

If you've found yourself here, that's a good thing. More and more people are moving forward with a more healthy and natural approach to their lifestyles. To reveal your inner curl is not a trend: it's an eco-friendly fashion-forward lifestyle choice. Once you learn how to treat your curls properly, you will never go back.

Seeking help through social media can result in information overload; sometimes actually picking up a good read or self-help book (remember those days?) is a better approach. If you've chosen *The ABCs*, you're sure to find it beneficial in your journey to be curly. I've done my best to share what I've learned through my training in curls and experience to help you find your way, curl friend!

My motivation in writing *The ABCs* is my clients. My "curl coaching sessions" at my studio have become so popular that I realized it was time to create a book to help more curlies who don't live close enough to make an appointment with me. A curl coaching session is a one-on-one appointment with my new curly client and myself. It's not about a curly cut; I don't have to touch my shears at all to rock your curly world. It's all about teaching you how to change a few things in your routine, adding in a few tips and techniques, and retraining how to work with your God-given curl pattern. From that one appointment at the studio, my clients' curls and mindsets are dramatically changed. As my clients return for other services, I add to their knowledge of how to take care of their hair. So think of this guide as my one-on-one coaching session with you. The best part is you can read at home and not fly to Toronto to see me!

If you're new to discovering your curls, don't rush to find a curly stylist. I suggest you read this book first. Change your washing, conditioning and styling routines to start your hair on its journey to curl recovery, *then* try to find a curly stylist for a curly cut once you have the ABCs down.

Note: *There are no limits to this guide. You've invested in The ABCs, so do read it cover to cover. Although I've made divisions for washing, styling and caring for individual curl patterns, you may wish to try a routine suggested in another curl category, or pattern, that may work better for you. You might be a combination of curl patterns, so a routine for you could be a mix of techniques. I have learned that nothing is absolute in the curly world, and being narrow-minded in your approach to your curls, thinking "This or that is just for this or that particular curl pattern" is very limiting—every curl is different. You can take the same two curlies, for instance, and they may look as if they have the identical curl pattern, but their hair has totally different reactions to product applications and drying techniques. So with this in mind, be open curly minded, and see where it takes you.*

Curly changes won't happen overnight. To bring out the curl in you will take time and effort. I'll be reminding you of this throughout the book. If you look at how long you've been doing a certain routine with your curls, it will understandably take some undoing. If, for example, you decide to redo your kitchen, do you blink your eyes and it's done? Or maybe you're changing your eating habits and trying to get into shape. Does this happen overnight? Your curls and changes will be a process, and it's a time frame that I can't estimate since every single curly is different. But you have taken the first step here.

Your first task is to take a selfie. Date it and track your progress as you move through the chapters, from curl rehab, washing, conditioning and styling to drying your curls, sleeping curly, product knowledge and so much more. You'll be fascinated when you look back at your curl journey as you move toward always being curly and loving it!

About the Author

Curly hair expert and texture specialist Adina has never known anything other than being a curly stylist. Entering the hair and beauty industry in 2003, she began her curl expert journey after graduating from cosmetology school, starting her apprenticeship at a downtown Toronto salon in Yorkville. For the most part, this salon specialized in curly hair. Adina was fascinated by the uniqueness and specialized service of a salon dealing with curls—curls of all shapes, sizes and textures. She was bitten by the curly stylist bug and headed to the United States to embark on her curly education and certifications. When Adina stepped into the New York Salon for her first curly course, she had no idea where that step would take her.

Today, Adina has both of the highest-acclaimed curl-expert certifications. She is both Ouidad and Curlisto certified, and she also has three Deva achievements: Advanced, the Art of Texture; named Canada's first Deva Curl Coach in 2016; and became an educator for Deva in 2017. At the time of this book's first publication, her salon, Curly Girls Studio, is the only studio in North America offering both Ouidad and Deva techniques to clients. This unique distinction helped Curly Girls make it onto blogTO's list of "The top 10 salons for curly hair in Toronto" less than two years after opening. The boutique studio caters exclusively to curls, providing only naturally curly hair-related service—no relaxers, no perms, no blowouts—and has received accolades for Always Being Curly!

Many clients come in just for Adina's personalized curl coaching sessions. Client after client is amazed at what they learn during their sessions at the studio. Adina felt it was time to put together a curly reference guide to help all the curl friends she can. This is her way of reaching those of you whom she won't have the opportunity to meet face to face—she will touch your curly lives with *The ABCs* instead.

So sit back, kick up your feet and enjoy this one-on-one curl coaching session put to paper to help bring out the curl in you. This book will change the way you look at your hair one curl at a time. Start from the basic ABCs, and learn how to "Always Be Curly" and love it!

Chapter 1

Curl Pattern & Elasticity

What's your curl pattern? Identify your curl pattern by comparing to the curl pattern guide on the following page. If you have more than one curl pattern, don't be concerned. It is totally normal to have more than one curl pattern on your head! Identifying your curl pattern(s) will help you learn how to care for your hair in the following chapters. As you see, the wavy pattern starts on the left, and as you move from 1-4, the kinkiest curls are at the end. If you are the kinkiest of curls and can barely see a curl pattern, you will be in the 3-4s. But in time, with love and curly hair care, you will be able to narrow down your pattern so you'll know if you are an "a" or "b" or "c." In this book, *A* stands for "Always," *B* stands for "Be" and *C* stands for "Curly," but in the curly world, they stand for something different. What does this all mean? Well, at some point, a curl guideline was created to define curl patterns. Hair in this curl guideline is broken up into four categories that are pretty much standard in the curly world to help identify your curl pattern. Knowing your curl pattern (some of you may have multiple patterns on your head) will help you better understand the care and routine suggested for your specific curls. The following are the four basic categories:

1. Straight
2. Wavy
3. Curly
4. Kinky Curly

The categories are further broken down into As, Bs and Cs, describing the type of wave, curl or kinky curl.

Curly Pattern Guide

Straight	2 Wavy	3 Curly	4 Kinky Curly

| | 2A | 2B | 2C | 3A | 3B | 3C | 4A | 4B | 4C |

What you should know about the curl patterns:

- Hair patterns are more fragile as the curl gets tighter.
- As we move across the categories, from 1 to 4, each subsequent pattern will require more conditioner and less shampooing for optimal curl and curl encouragement.
- Chemicals and heat are more damaging, and the effects longer-lasting, as you move through the categories, especially for the 3 and 4 curl patterns.
- Hair growth can take four times longer to show in the 4 curl pattern. If we look at all the bends there are in that curl pattern as it grows out,

it takes significantly longer to see a full curl formation. But for a 2a, a wavy pattern, for example, the hair grows straight out with minimal bends, so with this curl pattern, visual hair growth is much quicker.

That's not to say, however, that there are not fragile textures in the 2s, or kinky curly girls who have hair that grows super-fast—there are always exceptions. But this is a generalization based on the curly mass majority to help you understand how to specifically deal with your pattern.

When we speak of curls, it's interesting to know that **elasticity** is primarily responsible for a curl's ability to hold a curl. Many things can affect curls' elasticity, including:

- using harsh shampoos
- using conditioners that are not moisturizing enough
- using conditioning products that are too heavy, or not applying the conditioner properly and evenly throughout your hair
- not leaving conditioner on long enough
- doing too many treatments (you can over-proteinize your hair)
- curling or flat ironing your curls to excess, or even in moderation
- having chemical services done, such as perms, relaxers or straightening systems
- making poor choices for hair coloring/highlighting applications
- smothering hair with oils and serums (too much oil is counterproductive to hair growth and healthy curls)
- blow-drying
- using hair spray and styling products that contain alcohol
- not applying styling products properly

All of these products, services and habits can affect curls' elasticity and ability to hold a curl. Your curls have amnesia. They have forgotten who they are. This book will remind them.

This book has a chapter dedicated to helping your curls recover from each of the factors listed above. There, you'll learn how to turn around your routine to restore the elasticity, where possible. In certain situations, curls can be damaged beyond the point of no return and the elasticity can't be restored. Usually, this damage is caused from chemical straightening or relaxing, or excessive hot ironing or blow-dry service. In these cases, the curls must be grown out or cut off. You can grow out this damage, trimming ends little by little until all the damage has been cut off, or do a "big chop" instead, which involves taking the curly bull by the horns (or not-so-curly ends) and chopping off your hair, removing all the damaged hair and starting fresh. The resources in *The ABCs* will help you establish good routines to get the best from your new growing curls, if the big chop is what you feel needs to be done.

As you learn the new routines recommended here and your hair gets healthier, the elasticity will come back to your curls. At first you may feel your hair isn't growing. Why? Because you're getting more spring in your hair as you restore its elasticity. More curl bounce means more shrinkage in the length of your curls. When the elasticity has been restored as much as can be, you'll see the growth. If you're a kinky curly 4 pattern type and you've been shampooing a lot, you may feel you have never seen hair growth at all. This is because your hair needs more moisture provided by conditioner and less shampooing than any other curly hair pattern. Your shampooing routine has had your curls breaking off at the ends. You'll see your hair as being very dull, and there will be flakes on your hair that are not dandruff but instead hair breakage—hair dust!!! You may not have seen true hair growth your whole curly life! Your kinky curly pattern may more resemble a steel wool pad. Give your curls time and TLC (Tender Love & Conditioner), and you'll see your curl pattern emerge as you restore the moisture to your ever-so-thirsty curls. I have personally witnessed this, and it's amazing to see the transition.

Elasticity Test

The next time you wash your hair, do a simple test to check its elasticity. Pluck a wet single strand from your scalp from five areas of your head. One strand each from either side of your head (between the temple and the ear), one from the top of your head (crown), one each from the nape and your bangs. Write down where you pulled each strand from. The hair should be able to stretch up to 50 percent without breaking when wet, and only 20 percent when dry. Grab both ends and wrap the hair strand around your index fingers (if the length allows) and gently pull, as you would an elastic band.

If you pull the hair and it stretches without breaking, that's good. But what you're also looking for is whether the hair goes back to the same curl it had before you stretched it. If it doesn't, you have poor elasticity. If your curls break, that means you have very poor elasticity left in your hair, or possibly none at all. The results explain why your curls start out lovely when first washed, but then lose their bounce and drop, and are dry and frizzy within hours. There is no elasticity in your hair to hold that curl. You'll also be identifying where your hair may be the driest, with minimal elasticity resulting from:

- using shampoo or shampooing too often
- poor conditioning routines
- not leaving enough moisture/conditioner in your hair as your curl pattern dictates
- not leaving conditioner on long enough
- chemical services and excessive use of hot tools

   Note: A 2-step curl routine will be beneficial. First, do a protein treatment, and after you have rinsed out the treatment, follow with a hydrating conditioner to lock in the proteins. This will help strengthen the hair from the inside out and help restore its elasticity.

Another result to consider is if the test strand has little to no stretch at all; that means your curls are low in moisture/hydration. Moisturizing deep treatments should be added to your weekly or bi-weekly routine as needed.

The reason you should check five areas of your head of curls is to also establish whether you need to pay special attention to spots where the elasticity is more compromised than others. For example, you may find that there is no curl or poor elasticity at the side sections around the ear. This could be the result of tugging hair back and securing it in an elastic or hair tie. You would therefore have to pay special attention to that area and change that routine, perhaps by using clips to gently hold your hair back rather than elastics. Some curlies may find they have three or four different patterns on their head, so the elasticity test will show which sections may need extra hydration. I find that many times the crown area is the driest; therefore, the curl pattern is distorted with poor elasticity, owing to the difference in texture. You must be mindful of the conditioning needs of certain curl patterns on your head. The corkscrew and kinky patterns of the 3s and 4s need more moisture, achieved by using richer conditioners all over, but especially on the crown. For example, conditioner should be allowed to process the appropriate amount of time (two to three minutes, or whatever is recommended on the product label), and not be rinsed down the drain when you turn your back to the shower stream. A shower cap put on after you apply conditioner will help in this instance. Restore the moisture balance to your curls and you'll restore the elasticity.

The "Washing & Conditioning" chapter goes into more depth for your routine, but following is a very brief breakdown of washing habits for the curl patterns 2 to 4, or wavy to kinky curly curls.

Curl Pattern "2s" who have *fine wavy hair* will rinse all the conditioner from your hair. Leaving any in will weigh it down. Lightweight conditioners or cream rinses are great for your curl pattern. You'll have better success with lighter-weight products for styling, such as foams and mousses. You can use a light leave-in product or a spray gel to smooth over the outer layer of your hair to control frizz. If you have *coarse or thick wavy hair,* you'll be able to stretch your wash days more than those with fine wavy curl patterns. To control the dryness of your waves, you can leave some conditioner in your hair for moisture or use a leave-in conditioner. You can use a thicker, heavier styling product to support the coarse and dry wavy curl pattern to encourage your curls. But you can also apply a lightweight foam or mousse last, as a layering product, to encourage the most curl and control frizz. Compared to other patterns, wavy curls seem to be the most popular category of curl that people use hair sprays on. Try to use a pump hair spray and not an aerosol; butane in aerosol can be drying. If possible, opt for alcohol-free hair spray or try an alcohol-free spray gel as a finishing spray. Allow your waves and curls to dry completely before touching to reduce the frizz.

Curl Pattern "3s" should, in most cases, leave a little conditioner in your hair when doing the final rinse. You would do well with a leave-in styling product, styling cream or gel, or a combination of leave-in and gel. "Co-washing" (using your conditioner as a shampoo) is suggested; you can alternate between conditioner and shampoo to minimize the amount of natural oils being stripped from your curls from the washing routine. Most 3s wash with shampoo once a week and co-wash the other times. If you're a sporty curly, wet down and co-wash as much as you like, just minimize the frequency of shampoo.

Curl Pattern "4s" should engage in minimal shampooing frequency. As much as your hair screams for moisture and is dry, don't be tempted to smother it with oils and concoctions with castor oil. Condition, condition, condition is the name of the curly game for your pattern. Optimal is to wash your curls every three weeks with a shampoo, if you need to. Co-wash with a good conditioner or wet down your hair as much as you want. You will always leave conditioner in, as well as use a leave-in conditioner; oils are only to be applied as a light layer, to seal in a good conditioner or leave-in conditioner. A richer, more moisturizing product with a good slip is your requirement. "Slip" refers to a product's ability to slide on the hair. It's generally characterized by a loose or lighter styling product, sometimes a cross between a gelatinous texture and clear or milky consistency. Always layer your products properly, and no cocktails, kinky girl! Being lazy—pouring all your products in your hand, doing a one-step application—is going to get less-than-optimal results. Layer your products properly to maximize the benefits of each individual product you apply. The best way to layer your products for your curls is in this order: detangler, leave-in conditioner, styling cream, followed by sealing in your products with alcohol-free gel or lightly with oil.

> *Note: When referring to a "leave-in," it's not necessarily just leaving in your conditioner; it's a product specifically designed and labeled to be used as a leave-in conditioner. However, some conditioners have great ingredients in their formulations and can therefore be used as a leave-in. When I use the word "shampoo," I'm referring to sulfate-free products, of course.*

What is a good conditioner? A good conditioner is full of rich, non-stripping or non-drying ingredients such as silicones or oils; botanical ingredients such as panthenol, B5 and aloe vera; and proteins such as wheat, soy and quinoa. These are good key ingredients. The right conditioner is probably the most important product for any curly moving forward. Removing sulfates from your shampoo is key, too, but conditioner is the last thing applied and/or left in your hair before the styling products. So your base product, *conditioner*, needs to provide the proper moisture to your curls. Your next task will be to find a conditioner that works well for you, especially you tighter curlies in the 4 category who are using conditioner as a co-wash (again, meaning using conditioner as a shampoo, instead of actual shampoo, to keep curls hydrated to the max) and leaving conditioner in the hair. Some conditioners will leave a milky film. Sometimes this is a result of the curls not being wet enough when you leave your conditioner in, but most of the time it's the conditioner itself that is leaving curls flaky. Again, finding the correct conditioner is key.

Healthy hair is shiny hair? Not always. Don't be discouraged if you have a tighter curl pattern in the 3s or 4s and you don't ever see a shine in your hair. Just because your hair doesn't shine, it doesn't mean the curls are unhealthy. The hair diameter from wavy to extremely curly is very different. A wavy pattern with fewer bends has more of a flat area on the surface of the hair on which light can reflect, and therefore will show a shine. The tighter the hair, the less flat surface area there is for light to reflect on. Curl definition and good spring in your curls is far more important than shine, so keep this in mind during your curl journey.

What do all these curl patterns have in common? They all hate frizz! It's the curly hair mystery or curse! Hair with poor elasticity usually has a high frizz factor. Frizzy hair contributes to tangles, tangles contribute to excessive shedding. Learning how to get your hair to a healthy, happy curly state by knowing how to take care of your curls from start to finish and from the inside out is key. Fortunately, *The ABCs* will show you how. The next chapter deals with frizz. By identifying the cause of frizz, we can overcome and control it.

Chapter 2

Frizz!

Do you know how great it is to be on vacation on a tropical island wearing my little curls down and controlled, and not looking like a big, frizzy puffball? By the end of the beach day, most curlies are hiding under their hats; then, when dressing for dinner, they've flat-ironed their curls to a straight submissiveness to pretend their hair is anything but what it is—curly! Some curlies, on the other hand, are adorned with a massive puffball on their heads (reminds me of the fuzzy troll I used to have on my pencil when I was little), wandering around on holiday, telling themselves and everyone around them, "This is just what my curls do in hot climates." Remember Monica from *Friends*? The whole episode took place in Barbados. Yeah, that's not a good look, even for a star. I'm telling you right now, you don't need to have a bad curly hair day in hot climates! There may be seasons or climates that your curly hair likes better, but bad curly days will be a thing of the past as you learn how to care for your hair.

In fact, I welcome the humidity, dance in the ocean mist and fear not the rain. I'm fairly athletic: I kick-box and play beach volleyball for hours in the sun, but I never worry my hair will be "crazy way out there." I live my life not according to my curls, not hiding from adventures, but embracing them as I have embraced my curls. I'm not saying I never have any frizz or flyaways. That's part of being curly and my curls' personality. But I have a nice curl pattern and healthy ends, and that's most important to me when I'm in situations like vacationing or participating in sports. For the most part, my hair is controlled, not controlling me. My goal with *The ABCs* is getting you to enjoy your life and not be a slave to your curls' behavior and appearance, even on holidays. Are you ready to take control of your curls?

Every curly knows this word and hates it—frizz! Even the word makes you scowl at the thought of it, right? What causes frizz? How can you fight it?

The basic understanding of what you're trying to control is key to good curls. It's all about the routine: not using shampoo with sulfates, shampooing less and conditioning more, and knowing the goal is to control those little cuticles. Yes, it's as simple as that. A lot of forces affect those little critters (cuticles), but they can be controlled: to what level will depend on you and what you put in or take out of your curly hair routine to see what your hair is capable of achieving. Curly hair despair stops here! The amount of curly rehab time that's needed will be according to how naughty you've been to your curls and the effort you're willing to put in when implementing your new curly routines.

The "cortex" is the underlying layer fed from the hair bulb, so good hair starts from the root—healthy body and nutrition. What you use on the outside of your body affects cuticles, too. Here are just some of the factors affecting the hair strand, inside and out: the weather elements (heat and cold); excessive heat from hair dryers and styling tools such as flat irons; chemical services (color, highlights, relaxers or perms); heat from furnaces inside the home; illness and medication; changes in life such as aging and having babies; change of seasons; hard water; and hair products and routines.

Don't get overwhelmed, thinking, "Oh my gosh, 100-plus pages to know!" Should you feel this way, check out the "KISS" chapter and see how easy it is—10 steps, it's that simple! But you have to first understand why your curls are behaving the way they are to understand how to change your routine. So take a deep breath and take baby steps. Absorb and incorporate whatever you can into your routine at whatever pace you can as you move forward with curly rehab, and add steps as you get more comfortable. As the saying goes, Rome wasn't built in a day, and a lifetime of doing whatever you've been doing to your curls cannot be undone in a day either!

Hair grows out of the follicle at the root, your scalp, and down along each curly strand there are thousands of overlapping cuticles (depending on your hair length). The cuticles, when raised up, are what you observe as frizz. For example, think of shingles on the roof of a house and how they overlap down each side. The goal is to use proper shampooing and conditioning routines and products (or not to use certain products), and learn the proper application methods to keep those cuticles down, and thus control the frizz.

Cuticle

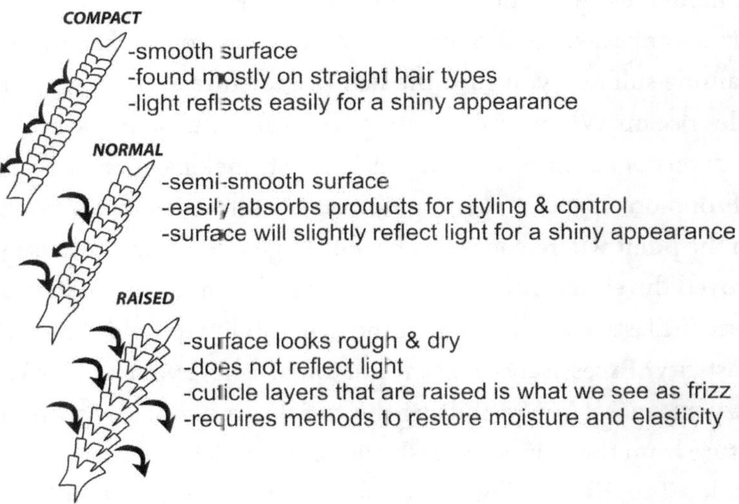

Note: *See Chapter 7, "Styling Your Curls—Porosity" (p. 82) for more information on the cuticle.*

When hair is very dry or dehydrated, your cuticle layer will be raised, because your curls and each raised cuticle ("shingle") are looking for moisture. Excessive heat, whether from weather or using styling irons, will raise the cuticle. Humidity will raise the cuticle.

Heat, we learned in high school chemistry, expands. Do you remember the metal ball and ring test from science class? As we heated the metal ball with the Bunsen burner, the ball would get bigger, and would no longer fit through the metal ring. So, with this concept in mind, when the warmer weather is upon us, our hair fibers expand as well, and a cuticle that is not properly hydrated and has been abused with hot irons will rise up, looking for moisture. Similarly, when chemical services are done, the active ingredients (such as ammonia) also cause the cuticle to rise; over-processed hair will have a high frizz factor, too, with little cuticles raised to the sky, seeking moisture. The cuticle, the frizz you see, seems to never go down because of the hair's overexposure to chemicals during color, straightening or perming processes.

So in the summer, when it's hot outside, if your hair isn't hydrated properly, those numerous little cuticles running all the way down each hair strand will rise up toward heaven and look for moisture. When you use harsh shampoos containing sulfates, you strip the hair of moisture and, no surprise, the cuticles rise up. When you're heating your hair with flat irons, hot combs, blow-dryers or curling irons, you are, in effect, cooking your curls at 200 to 400°F, or more. If you're a curling-iron or flat-iron user, you may eventually reach the point where you won't be able to go curly at all, because you've destroyed the elasticity in your hair. Remember you learned in the "Curl Pattern & Elasticity" chapter that the hair's ability to hold a curl is based on elasticity? Excessively using any hot tool will have your hair looking like a frizzy hot mess! You're abusing the cuticle even more by stripping the moisture from the hair with harsh chemical services such as highlighting and color. Top that all off with excessive washing, because your hair seems to never look good for more than a few hours, if at all, when you go curly. It's time to get off that vicious cycle that always leads to bad curly hair days! By learning the correct steps (methods and routines) and product applications, you can control and reduce the frizz factory production on your curly head.

You must consider your washing routines when wanting to control the cuticle, the frizz. Shampoos with sulfates really aggravate the cuticle. Sulfates are harsh cleansers and are too aggressive an ingredient to use on your curls. These shampoos clean so well that they raise the cuticle to a point that, in most cases, it will no longer go down. The sulfates are designed to lift the cuticle and remove the dirt, debris, styling product and natural oils from your scalp. But for a curly, these sulfates are too harsh and typically result in the hair becoming squeaky clean and dehydrated. Throw in an ineffective conditioner and you're frizzy before you even style your hair. When you shampoo with sulfates, this ingredient always remains in your hair. When the shampoo is extremely harsh (some shampoos are harsher than others), the sulfates strip the hair, making curls thinner, finer and dry. Squeaky clean hair is bad. Shampoos that create this feel have stripped your hair of protective nourishing oils. *So when I say the squeaky clean feeling you like is bad, it's BAD!* All the natural oils have been stripped, leaving hair lifeless and lackluster. When hair is left in a dehydrated state, its elasticity is affected. If you've affected the elasticity of the hair, the curl pattern is affected. As explained earlier, elasticity contributes to the hair's natural ability to curl and hold its curl. It's a vicious cycle you're on. And it's time to break the cycle.

Healthy hair that has a good balance of moisture and elasticity (from not being stripped by sulfates in shampoos such as clarifiers or chelating shampoos) will have better curl retention and reduced frizz factor. That's a lot of benefit from changing step one of your routine. By adding a few more recommendations, you'll be rocking your waves and curls in no time.

Some luxury brands sold at salons have key ingredients to counteract the effect of the sulfates and are therefore not as harsh. Using a conditioner that's very moisturizing balances out the effects of the sulfates. Some curlies may opt to stay with these brands. Really, it's just a matter of trial and error for some of you. Shampooing frequency makes a big difference, too.

Shampooing less often will result in less stripping of the oils and drying out the cuticles. But if you want a more guaranteed result, sulfate-free is a better choice.

For the record, retail brands have jumped on the sulfate-free bandwagon. I find it funny that some brands have opted to put "sulfate-free" on the conditioner of the partnering shampoo. A sulfate is a cleansing agent not found in conditioners. There shouldn't be sulfates in conditioner. Ever. At least, this is not an ingredient used in a conditioning formula I've ever heard of. Using this word on a conditioner bottle is just a marketing ploy to get consumers' attention.

In order to stay on track, I can't list all the good, the bad and the ugly ingredients in various shampoos here; you'll have to do this research for your curls yourself. If a bottle says sulfate-free, you'll have to read the other ingredients to make sure there isn't another one that strips the hair, making up for the lack of sulfates. There are also applications online that you can download that will actually break down the products and ingredients for you.

Step one in changing your routine is the shampoo. If you start off wrong there, it's all downhill with your curls. Your curls won't even have a chance to show you their true potential if you don't change your shampoo, especially if you wash your hair frequently. We'll move on to "Curl Rehab" next so you'll learn how to better care for your curls. As you make your way through the following chapters, you'll discover methods and routines to help control and reduce the frizz factor. Guaranteed!

Curl Story

As described in the "Curl Pattern & Elasticity" chapter, hair becomes more fragile as you move across the curl-pattern categories, with 4 being the most fragile. Until my daughter was 10 years old, she had very straight hair (she began to get a wave in her pre-teens). Her cuticles were so compact thanks to her hair pattern, which was bone-straight, no bends at all, that she could use the harshest of shampoos without affecting her cuticles. She was young—though growing at the speed of light—and her hair was more resilient. Once she began to get the wave in her hair, however, it became a totally different story! Her hair began showing signs of frizz, so I switched her to sulfate-free shampoo, and she and her waves are as happy as can be.

Chapter 3

Curl Rehab

Welcome to your curl rehab! Hair despair stops here and curl recovery begins today! You have decided to embrace your curls and not fight them any longer. Here you'll find the steps to get you on the right track!

Most curls have to work at curl recovery, especially if you have chemical damage from straightening systems, perms, excessive highlights or color processes; you're a product junkie, smothering and suffocating your curls in oil, or always blow-drying your hair and killing your curls with your double-barreled flat iron blasted to 450-plus degrees! Or maybe you're washing your hair too frequently and styling it wrong. Oh, those poor little curls! It's a shame what all those tender curls have been subjected to. Let's review the naughty list and take a sneak peek into the simple steps and remedies below. I will expand on the remedies in the chapters that follow. For now, let's just take baby steps to get you into the curly groove.

Do you:

1. Use sulfate shampoo? Then change to sulfate-free shampoo.

2. Apply hair oils such as olive, coconut, argon, Moroccan and castor oil, and find your curls are flat and dehydrated, and there's a hazy film left on the outer layer? Then clarify the buildup and start fresh (see the "Washing & Conditioning" chapter under clarifying).

3. Find your hair is frizzy and your curls are not defined when you try to go curly after having straightened your hair for months or years? Know that one flat-iron session can affect your hair, depending on curl pattern, for a month or even more! Have you noticed your hairline is receding or there are straight, straggly pieces that never curl anymore around your face when you try to go curly? FYI, your front hairline is very fragile—the most fragile area on your head of curls. Or maybe when you try to go curly it's a hot frizzy mess! What you've done is destroyed the elasticity in your hair and it will take time to get it back or grow it out. The solution? Don't do it! And of course read *The ABCs* to help you change your ways with washing and styling, and let the styling tips guide your curl rehab.

4. Blow-dry your hair? In general, it's less damaging to the curls than curling irons and flat irons, but again, depending on the texture and strength of your hair, it can be just as bad as the hot iron. The solution? Don't do it! But if you do blow-dry on occasion, make sure you use a heat protectant before the heat is applied to buffer some of the damaging effects. Do moisturizing treatments the next wash to help bring the curl back and restore the elasticity. You need to reconsider your styling options and perhaps try a roller set to alter your curl pattern in a healthier, less damaging way.

5. Try to be curly and use your blow-dryer to diffuse your curls, but your curls get all frizzy and the curl just doesn't hold? In the "Drying Your Curls" chapter, you'll learn how to diffuse properly. In the "Washing & Conditioning" and "Styling Your Curls" chapters, you'll learn how to restore the elasticity with your washing, conditioning and styling product application so your hair holds the curl better.

6. Use products on your curls but are not sure which product to apply first? You'll find the answers in the "Product Knowledge" chapter.

7. Expose your curls to aggressive chemical services (perms, relaxers, straightening systems)? You need to get off this over-processing train! The solution sometimes involves either a big chop or painfully growing out your hair and finding protective styles to close the gap on the fresh new roots and processed ends. The "Washing & Conditioning" chapter will get your new roots and natural hair on track.

8. Apply poor-quality hair color and application methods? Home color is sometimes what curlies have to do, but make sure you buy the best-quality products and use them the correct way. Refer to the "Color & Highlighting" chapter, with tips and techniques to guide you.

9. Have little baby hairs that never seem to grow around your face? Check out the "Curl Bits" chapter for info on that curly dilemma.

10. See little or no visible hair growth at all? You need to revamp all your routines with almost all the lessons in this book!

I could add a lot more to this naughty curly list, but you get the message. In the following chapters, you'll find answers to a lot of your concerns and some things you may never have even thought of that will help you be curly and love it.

In a nutshell, however, the more naughty and abusive you've been to your curls, the longer it will take to bring them back to a healthy state. Don't get discouraged, it's worth it! You've come to the right place to learn how to start your curl recovery. Although it won't happen overnight, the benefits you will see will far outweigh the time you have to invest. This chapter is just a glimpse into curl recovery. Changing what you use to wash your hair as well as your washing routines, and slowly weaning from constantly stripping your scalp of natural oils are key. It could take a month or longer to see the full benefits of these changes, so be patient. Keep in mind that if you are a flat-iron junkie with straight, straggly pieces everywhere or, more specifically, your bangs because you have flat-ironed them over and over and over to smooth them, you will more than likely have to grow out your hair and trim your ends little by little. You can create finger coils and curls on the straight ends to help match curl pattern; it may save you from chopping off the bangs until you grow enough curly length. If you find your hair has receded, well that is between you and God as to whether it can be restored. Generally, abuse to that fragile hairline is permanent.

So if you're committed to the ABCs and put aside your iron, don't slip (most of my flat-iron junkies slip once). As I mentioned before, you will do one month's worth of damage to your curls from that single use. Just imagine the wonderful potential your frizz-laden, flat and broken curly mane has if you never look back on the 450-plus-degree burning double barrel! The ugly duckling curly phase will pass. Be patient!

As for you curlies who have been getting perms or relaxer (hidden curls in disguise), you will have to grow out the damage or do the big chop. You can do braids, being mindful not to have them too tight around the hairline. Don't change one bad styling habit for another. There are twist and finger coils you can do to blend the straightened hair to the natural curl as it grows out. Headbands and scarves at the hairline will hide the transition line when you're just starting the natural growing-out process.

You should all do weekly treatments to expedite the process and growth, but don't turn to hair oils, slathering them everywhere in an attempt to add moisture to your curls in recovery. That said, if oil is your thing, use light varieties like jojoba (which is closest to our natural sebum, or what our scalp creates), coconut, macadamia or avocado oil; do not use olive oil unless it is pure—not a generic olive oil brand from the bulk or box stores. That kind of oil is not even good for cooking! But I'll save the cooking oil lecture for the cookbook. Curls need to breathe to recover, not suffocate under oil. Oils are for your scalp, not the curly strands. Scalp massages are also highly recommended.

As a transitioning flat-iron curly, don't get discouraged if you see great curls when you first style your hair, but as the day goes on your curls don't remain as perky. You have been ruining the elasticity in your hair for months, maybe years. You need the elasticity restored for your curls' memory to help hold the curl. If the damage is not extensive, the hair will learn how to retain ("remember") the curl with TLC: Tender Love & Conditioner. Sulfate-free shampoo, shampooing less and adding treatments to your routine will help. If you have pushed your hair past its limit, you will have to grow out your hair to see your curl pattern in its full glory with the new growth.

What if you wear a ponytail or headband, or you're a curly who is a styling junkie, applying gels or hair spray to smooth back the hair? When you try to wear your hair curly and not pulled back, you then might ask, "Why is my curl dropping after initially getting a great styling result the first few hours after washing or maybe just the first day?" Here's the deal: Pulling back the hair in this fashion has compromised the elasticity in your hair. Remember, elasticity contributes to the ability of the hair to hold its curl. It will just take time to restore the elasticity that has been continually stretched out. Condition well and do light treatments. Once this happens, your hair will hold its curl. Try using a styling foam or spray gel on the straight pieces, as this sometimes helps to encourage the curl better without weighing it down with heavier styling products. However, if you have thick, wavy hair, its own weight may not give you the best second-day hair; you may get more favorable results if you use a gel or other stronger holding styling product that will keep the curl better. And seek out a curly stylist who specializes in cutting techniques to remove weight, not a regular stylist who will use thinning shears or randomly texturize the hair.

As you can see we have a lot to cover. So let's move into the meat and potatoes of curly rehab and expand on the above with the "Washing & Conditioning" chapter to get your curls on the right track. Remember, Rome wasn't built in a day, nor will your hair change overnight. All good things take patience, time and effort.

Chapter 4

Washing & Conditioning

If you've decided to read this book, you're likely already aware of changing your shampoo to a sulfate-free brand instead of the regular sulfate-laden ones. But in case you haven't heard, know that this ingredient is not curl-friendly. Sulfates are ingredients that are very harsh on the hair strands, especially those that are curly. The more bends there are in the hair, or the finer the texture, the harsher this ingredient is on a curly-textured person compared to a straight-haired friend. Sulfates are found in products like dishwasher detergent and laundry soaps. That can't be good for hair, especially fragile curls! Curly hair needs moisture and does not do well when stripped of all its natural oils. Sulfates strip the strands of much-needed moisture and leave hair dehydrated.

Some of the harsher shampoos can even thin hair, making strands straggly and the diameter of the strand finer. Sulfates also leave a residue that is never completely rinsed out when shampooing. When you decide to make a change in shampoo, trying to get used to less-bubble, or in some cases no-bubble, shampoo is hard. Not having that squeaky, what-you-think-is-clean feeling is a hard habit for most curlies to break. We have been conditioned for years, dating back to the 1930s, that we should clean our hair frequently. In the '60s, you were considered a hippie if you didn't wash your hair frequently, every day. Even today, commercials are airing with girls washing their hair as camera angles show lots of lather all over their heads. The hair model is oohing and aahing as she washes her bubbly hair. The commercial ends with a professional model (after a styling crew has blow-dried, flat-ironed and smeared her hair with oil and hair spray) with long, flowing, smooth and bouncy locks, all aimed to convince you that your hair will be the same by sudsing up. Well, get ready for a change! Drop the shampoo with sulfates from your routine. The benefits of going sulfate-free far outweigh the initial adjustment you may have to go through for a short time as you change your shampoo addiction.

As a curly newbie altering your shampooing routine, you may find that your scalp will go through various stages as you wean yourself off the sulfate shampoos, so try to slowly cut down the washing frequency. For as long as your scalp has known a routine, it has been continually stripped of its natural oils. Don't be surprised, therefore, if your scalp begins to flake and you feel these crusty-like greasy layers and scales on the scalp. The sebaceous glands (responsible for creating the natural oils that moisturize the roots of your hair) will take a little time to normalize and get used to creating natural oils at a rate associated with your new washing pattern. This adjustment period can last anywhere from one to four weeks, maybe more. Just be patient and your scalp will adjust. If you must rinse your hair more often to remove the flakes and buildup you may experience, that's fine. Try to resist, however, the temptation to wash with shampoo every day. Moving forward, once you reduce your frequency of using sulfate shampoo, switching to a sulfate-free shampoo is your next step. Some of you may opt to go cold turkey and just jump right in with the no-sulfate shampoo routine. Be aware that even sulfate-free shampoos have cleansing ingredients that strip the scalp and curly strands, so you really want to minimize the number of times you are washing your hair and scalp in general. Try to find your own comfort level and balance, keeping all this in mind. These recommendations do not take priority over seeing a doctor if you are concerned about your scalp.

As you may recall from the beginning of the book, I said, **"Wash less and condition more!"** For years, I have been teaching my extremely curly clients to wash less (usually about once every three to four weeks) and condition more. That means those with the kinky curly pattern will "co-wash" all the other times she wets down her hair. This non-shampoo cleansing routine is referred to as the co-wash method, or simply washing your hair with conditioner. Co-washing is something you may incorporate permanently into your routine after you wean from shampoo. You can wet down your hair as often as you like, cutting out shampoo from your routine. Just know that you will have to go through the styling product application routine each time you wet down your hair.

After years of telling 3- and 4-pattern clients not to shampoo, I decided to take it one step further and have gone *100 percent shampoo-free*. I have cut out shampoo altogether and only co-wash. The end result is amazing. When I first cut out shampoo, my curl pattern was 2b—now it's closer to a 3. I used to shed excessively: handfuls of hair would be all over my hands every time I shampooed. Since going shampoo-free, I have a lot less hair shedding and the texture of my curl is much smoother. Another amazing thing I've noticed is I get better day-after curl! And my hair's elasticity is much better. Remember what I said, *"The hair's ability to hold a curl is all based on elasticity."* Going cold turkey with shampoo has resulted in a fantastic curl benefit list any curly would be happy to call her own!

Consider going shampoo-free if you're game. It's all about finding the right conditioner. I first tried an organic brand, but it didn't feel as though my scalp and hair were clean. The second one I tried for a couple of weeks was tea tree oil-based; my scalp felt clean, but the conditioner itself was very heavy on my hair and made my curls look floppy. Then I began using a medium-weight conditioner with mint as one of its ingredients, and it is what I still use today. It works perfectly for me. I feel that using a mint-based conditioner cleans and clarifies my scalp and breaks down the excessive oil and styling-product buildup, so I don't have the need to shampoo. Mint as an ingredient is key!

Steps to cleansing your scalp with sulfate-free shampoo or co-washing:

1. Use warm water and stimulate the scalp with your fingertips to massage your natural oils and break them down (washing with cold water will not break down the oils).
2. Do not be aggressive with the mid-shaft and ends of your curls; rub them between your palms; or scrub your curls as you would a pot or pan.
3. Apply your shampoo (or conditioner, if choosing the co-wash method) along your fingertips and use circular motions to cleanse and stimulate the whole scalp, from the nape of your neck, around your ears to the front hairline.
4. Next, gently scrunch the ends of your curls up to the roots to spread the cleansing product.
5. Thoroughly rinse out the product buildup and dirt from your scalp.
6. Apply your conditioner as the next step if you're using sulfate-free shampoo, or reapply your conditioner if you're co-washing.

Note: When you co-wash, you're washing with conditioner. The first application of the conditioner gets rinsed out, just as you would with shampoo, because it will contain styling product, debris and oils from your scalp. So if you have a curl pattern that requires leaving in conditioner, the second application of the conditioner will be on clean hair.

What if you thought it was good to wash hair with cooler water? When washing your curls, start with warmer water. This will help dissolve the natural oils and break down some of the product buildup before you shampoo or co-wash. If you use colder water to wash your hair, you won't break down the oils. Think of when you wash a greasy pan. If you pour cold water in the pan, it will harden the oils and the pan won't get clean, even with the dish soap. Warm water, however, heats up the oil and loosens it.

Feel free to rinse with cooler water after you condition the hair if you find it works better for you, but definitely wash your curls in warmer water.

As I have mentioned before (a few times), the key to a successful co-wash (not using shampoo as often or at all to wash your hair) is finding the right conditioner. I opt for mint-based conditioners, as the mint helps to break down the oils and stimulate the scalp. Your co-wash product searching will be up to you and your scalp to figure out what works best. Do make sure you give the conditioner a good try, not just one use before judging its effectiveness. You should try up to a couple of weeks, depending on how often you co-wash, to see if it's the correct conditioner for you. Just when you think you have it figured out, the season changes and you may have to search for a richer or lighter conditioner based on your curly season needs.

Co-Wash Tip for Drier, Tighter Textures

Try applying conditioner to your hair when it's dry and do a pre-detangle with your fingers before going into the shower. You can even let the conditioner sit on your curls for a few minutes beforehand. Then, when you go to wash your hair, let a little warm water trickle in slowly, raking your fingers through to allow the conditioner to deeply penetrate the strands' cuticles and continue to detangle your curls. Follow the rest of your steps for cleansing your scalp and ends as above.

Excessive Hair Shedding

If you're losing a lot of hair, increase the frequency of whichever cleansing routine you have chosen to go with. Sometimes with certain curl patterns, if you stretch the period between washing or rinsing times too far, you may find you tangle and have more knots than if you do a rinse or co-wash a little more often. We all naturally shed a certain amount of hair daily, but when you allow your hair to get too knotted, you'll be pulling out good hair (that is still attached to the root) with bad hair (the hair you have naturally shed) when you get to the detangling part of your routine. So unless you've done the finger-coil style, where the curls have been locked together, or a roller set, I find that for most curls, three or four days is optimal to do a wash, rinse down or co-wash. As with everything curly related, there are exceptions! At the opposite end of the time frame I've set out above, I've known some curlies with hair patterns from wavy to kinky curly with a dry or coarse texture who can go for 7 to 10 days without washing or co-washing with not even a wet down! Let your hair shedding and tangling be your guide, and test the time frame for what works best for you.

Curl Story

When I was a cosmetology student, our school provided hair services to clients a few days a week. Right at the beginning of my schooling, a girl in her mid-20s came in with the softest, most beautiful 3a curl pattern. Keep in mind, I never knew of the curly hair movement at that time. She brought in a picture of a cute bob and asked for her cut to be the same. Before I took her to the shampoo sink, she asked me not to use shampoo when washing her hair and to simply wet it down. She told me she never uses shampoo—*ever*! I thought it was a different approach back then. Her curl pattern was beautiful and healthy, and her scalp felt and looked clean. She always came to mind as I learned about curls. That's part of what inspired me to do the same years later.

If you're not going to follow my lead and never use shampoo, below are recommendations for the washing routine for curl patterns 1 to 4. Yes, 1 is straight hair, not curly, but just in case a straight-patterned person is reading this, I've included it as well. Please refer to the "Curl Pattern & Elasticity" chapter if you have not already determined what your curl pattern is.

Curl Patterns 1-2, Fine Hair

- Shampoo and condition two or three times a week.
- Rinse hair clean after applying your conditioner (leaving conditioner in will just weigh down your curls).

Curl Patterns 1-2, Coarse Hair

- Shampoo and condition once a week, and wet down or co-wash once a week.
- If you have dry, coarse, wavy curls, either leave some conditioner in or use a product marked as a leave-in conditioner.

Curl Pattern 3

- Shampoo and condition once a week.
- Co-wash every other time you wash your hair.
- Leave some conditioner (as much as 25 percent) in your hair every time to provide a nice moisture base for your styling product.

Curl Pattern 4

- Shampoo and condition: wash once every three to four weeks.
- Co-wash as many times as you need to and feed your hair conditioner; leave as much as 50 percent in.
- Yes, you read correctly: leave up to 50 percent of your conditioner in! Your curl pattern screams for moisture, so feed your craving curls conditioner.

Note: I said this before and I'll say it again—*Find the right conditioner!*

Conditioning Steps

The first thing to do when in the shower is start your hair routine before doing anything else. No washing your face, or shaving first. Get right to the curls!

1. Shampoo or co-wash your hair.
2. If you're co-washing as your first step, rinse out the conditioner as you would a shampoo to get rid of buildup and debris, and follow with your conditioner for the conditioning step.
3. Take a generous amount of conditioner and spread evenly all over the palms of your hands. Apply conditioner from mid-shaft to

ends. Apply any residue from roots grazing downward for equal distribution.

4. If you have shorter hair or fine hair, try not to apply conditioner on your scalp, as the conditioner may be too heavy and make your scalp greasy.

5. Run the conditioner down your hair strands with your fingers using a gentle gliding motion to make sure your curls are evenly coated with the moisture the conditioner is designed to provide.

6. Allow conditioner to process as instructed (usually 1-3 minutes).

7. Gently trickle water on your hair and squish it in. Add more conditioner if you feel it's needed; add a little more water and "squish to condish!" Keep scrunching until you feel your conditioner has thoroughly saturated your hair. The extra trickles of water really help the conditioner enter the hair shaft and dilute the larger molecules to allow for a deeper penetration for a better-hydrated cuticle.

8. After the conditioner has rested on your curls for the allotted time, you can detangle the hair with your fingers or wide-toothed comb. There are times when this curly stylist uses combs to detangle, so if that's your thing, use whichever method you believe is best for you and your curls.

9. Hair strands should feel hydrated and smooth if you have done this step properly. Do the "Cuticle Check" (p. 81), and if you still feel your hair is frizzy as you pinch down the strand, use the "Pinch & Glide Frizz Buster" method found in the "Styling Your Curls" chapter.

10. Rinse conditioner out according to your hair's needs. Wavys typically rinse clean, curly curls leave some conditioner in and kinky-curly types may leave some to all of the conditioner in for extra moisture.

Simply slapping a glob of conditioner on your hair and letting it sit a minute will not hydrate those thirsty curls. To get your curls in good condition, the conditioning step is really important. Take your time with this step and you will be creating a hydrated curly canvas that your styling products will glide over, which in turn will result in an amazing curly style.

> **Note:** *For low- and high-porosity hair or additional help dealing with excessive frizz, refer to "Styling Your Curls: Pinch & Glide Frizz Buster," and implement this method when doing your conditioning step.*

Conditioning for Varied Curl Patterns

Curly hair can grow in different thicknesses and densities on various areas of the head. You could, in fact, have multiple patterns. For example, I have one client who has a very loose wavy pattern on both sides of her head by her ears. Underneath, at the back by the nape of her neck, she has super-straight hair, while at the crown she has really tight curls. How you would handle this varied curly scenario is to go light on applying conditioner on the loose sides and nape, but make sure the crown is thoroughly coated with conditioner and covered with a shower cap while the conditioner processes for the product's recommended time according to its directions. Most curlies have a dehydration problem with their curls at the crown. Using a shower cap protects the conditioner from being rinsed out or diluted by the shower stream. Rinsing out your conditioner should be your last step in the shower. You should apply your conditioner where the hair is the curliest or driest first; for example, apply to the crown first if that's your driest area, then at the nape of your neck second and the sides of your head last. You may even want to have special conditioner that is a little richer for the crown for extra moisture if you have super-kinky curly dry hair in that area. Or apply a true leave-in conditioner in that area only.

Treatments

For dry curls, you need to make time for treatments to restore them and help keep the curls hydrated. Depending on your hair's texture, a treatment could be something you need to do once a week or once a month. Do you find you have no time to do a deep treatment in the shower because your schedule is so busy with work, school and family? Try fitting one in while making dinner. Apply a treatment or deep conditioner to dry curls *before* you head to the shower. It will give a little extra moisturizing time to your dehydrated curls. Or, if you have identified that your curls are really dry at the ends, but you have no time to hang in your shower while a treatment processes, simply wet the ends a few inches up from the bottom, apply treatment and cover the ends with a plastic bag. You can even use plastic wrap instead and let hair rest while you finish making dinner, do homework... whatever. You can put on a toque to create some heat on the ends, tucking them under the hat for deeper product penetration. Now that's multitasking! When ready to wash your curls, you can still shampoo or co-wash in the shower: just leave the ends until last to rinse while you cleanse your scalp. The final step is to rinse all your curls from roots to ends and seal with a good conditioner everywhere.

Also, busy curlies, aside from the multitasking method above, don't skip your weekly treatment if you find you don't have the time for a treatment with heat and/or processing time as required by the product label. A three-minute mini-treatment in the shower is better than holding off until you can do a fully processed treatment. Before you know it, weeks will have gone by without doing a treatment, waiting for the opportune time. Follow the product treatment label instructions as per application, except do a shorter processing time in the shower, gym or wherever you can fit it in. Usually deep treatments are once a week for very damaged hair. Processing time varies from usually 5 minutes to 20, or can be left on all night (but *only as instructed*). Let the dryness or health of your curls be your guide.

> **Note:** *Some textures of curls do not like protein treatments, or only like certain types of proteins (there's wheat-, soy-, quinoa-based, etc.); others only need protein treatments once in a while.*

You have to learn to *pay attention to your curls and what they are telling you.* Too many protein treatments can cause hair strands to become brittle. Be sure to use products as directed. That said, if you find you're not getting the results you want, either cut back the frequency recommended in the instructions or stop using it altogether. Your hair may not like the protein in the treatment you are using. Some hair, perhaps contrary to product instructions, processes better with heat, and others without. Also, don't think leaving a treatment on for an excessive amount of time will help. Do as directed—sometimes less is more. Doing treatments too often or leaving product on for excessive periods can *actually make hair drier.* "Over-proteinizing" the curls is not good! Again, follow directions, unless you're doing a modified "no time for treatment" three-minute one, as described above.

Clarifying

Do you find yourself thinking, "My hair is so awful, my curls feel heavy and are falling flat, and my hair looks dull?" Or maybe you're thinking that the gel you used to love is just not working anymore. Every curl needs a little clarifying once in a while to remove product buildup. Pollutants from the air that have settled on the hair, and oil and residue from certain products you may be using also cause this negative reaction. Clarifying to the rescue! I also mention this step in the chapter "Product Knowledge" under Clarifying or Chelating Shampoos. It's an easy solution to gently remove product buildup.

1. Prepare a mixture of 2 parts sulfate-free shampoo or conditioner to 1 part baking soda in a plastic cup.
2. Apply to wet hair, then scrunch from roots to ends to distribute; allow mixture to sit on your hair for a few minutes.
3. Add a little more warm water to spread the mixture throughout your hair.
4. Rinse clean.
5. Follow with your conditioner.

    Note: *Hair will be soft and feel smooth. Don't overdo this clarifying step, as it can strip too much moisture if done too frequently. Do once a month or as needed.*

Another option is apple cider vinegar. Some may find cider vinegar is very hard on the curls because of the acidity. But some people, using a spray bottle, will apply apple cider vinegar either straight or diluted with cooled boiled water to dampened hair, leaving it on for a few minutes, then rinsing clean. Some even use this formula to remove minerals from hard water or well-water mineral deposits. Test a small area, as with anything you plan to do on your head of curls, to see how your curls and scalp react. Do not use if you have any open sores or cuts on your scalp. If your test patch does well without any irritation, clarify your whole head of curls with apple cider vinegar, rinse clean and seal with conditioner. Vinegars tend to leave a slight smell on hair, even when rinsed well, whereas baking soda will not leave any residual odors.

At this point of your curl recovery, make sure you have:

1. Taken a selfie!
2. Clarified your hair (as directed above) to remove buildup from your curls as set out in "Washing & Conditioning."
3. Started using sulfate-free shampoo and good conditioner.
4. Completed the elasticity test, having checked the five areas of your head and recorded the results, so you know how to treat your hair when choosing your styling products and methods.

Now get ready for some "Product Knowledge" in the next chapter. You need to learn about products before you're taught how to apply them. You'll learn what different styling products do in order to help you decide what to use to get the best curly style.

Chapter 5

Product Knowledge

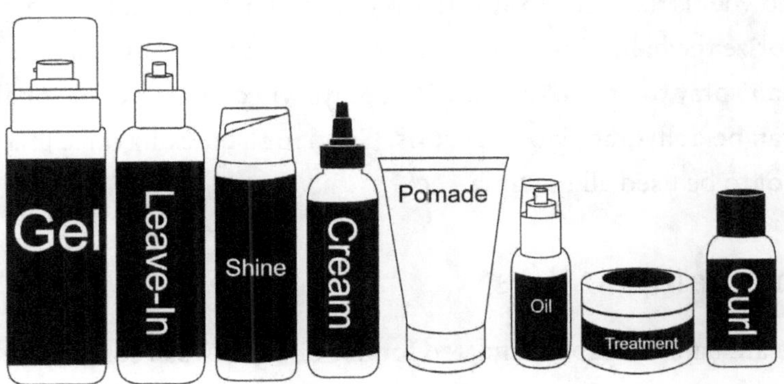

To get the right results for a truly rocking curly style, you need to know what the various products do so you can decide which are suitable for your curl pattern. I won't get into the chemistry, ingredients and formulations, as this would take over the whole book. It will be up to you to research and see what works best for your hair. Products and formulas are designed to work certain ways to achieve certain results. What you have learned in "Washing & Conditioning" and will learn in the "Styling Your Curls" chapter will ensure you know how to apply the products to make them work effectively. Your curly style results will let you know if they're the right products for you.

Shampoos

These clean the scalp and hair, removing the buildup of oils and styling product residue. For curlies, a sulfate-free shampoo is your best option. If using a sulfate-based product, limit the number of times you shampoo your hair per week. Excessive washing strips hair and scalp of moisture, resulting in a drier and finer texture of curls and with the elasticity ultimately compromised. **(Remember: The hair's ability to curl to its maximum potential and hold its curl is based on elasticity.)**

Dry Shampoos

These products usually come in a powder form and are sprinkled on the hair. The powder is designed to absorb the oil, and it may contain a fragrance to deodorize the hair. New to the market are spray shampoos that are applied like hair spray to dry up the oils. The sprays will contain butane or alcohol and can be dehydrating on the curls. Good for a quick fix once in a while, but not to be used all the time.

Hair Shampoo Bars

These are bars of soap formulated for use on hair. Make sure to check the ingredients, as some bars may contain the same drying ingredients to hair as those found in liquid shampoos, and will strip the hair of its much-needed moisture. Wet your hair and the shampoo bar, coating your fingertips with the soap; with your fingertips, massage the bar soap lather onto the scalp, and gather your hair by small handfuls, scrunching from the ends to the roots. Rinse your hair clean and finish with conditioner.

Co-Washes

There are some shampoos labeled as a co-wash. Co-washes can have bubbles or be lather-free. Most are a creamy consistency and sometimes contain oils in their formulation. Co-washes are supposed to be more hydrating than a traditional shampoo and can work on a variety of curls.

In the curly world, the term "co-wash," as previously mentioned, is actually using your conditioner as you would a shampoo.

Clarifying or Chelating Shampoos

These shampoos are intended to be used occasionally to remove buildup. Most are too harsh for curls and can leave hair a matted mess. A more economical and simpler option is to clarify with baking soda and sulfate-free shampoo, as mentioned in the "Washing & Conditioning" chapter. Some curlies opt to use apple cider vinegar to clarify or even remove minerals from hard water deposits. You can put pure apple cider vinegar in a spray bottle and mist on hair, let sit a few minutes and rinse clean. Some may find vinegars too acidic and therefore drying to the hair.

Cream Rinses / Instant Conditioners

These are generally very light conditioners intended to rinse clean. Cream rinses help detangle curls and are better for fine hair textures or wavy curls that are in good condition. Because these rinses and conditioners are light-weight, they don't weigh down your curls. Follow product instructions for how long it should be left on the hair before rinsing clean.

Conditioners

Available in a large variety of brands catering to many needs, some conditioners are heavily laden with oils to hydrate the curls after being washed. Shampoos are meant to cleanse, while the conditioner is meant to add moisture to the hair in varying degrees. As mentioned, some curlies use conditioners as a co-wash. Follow instructions, but usually conditioners need to be left on the hair for a few minutes to process in order for the curls to receive the benefits of the product and conditioning step. For drier, tighter curls in the 4s curl pattern, it's generally recommended to leave a little, some or even all the conditioner in the hair. The looser the curl, the less conditioner you would leave in.

Spray Leave-In Conditioners (Liquid)

These are very lightweight conditioners that can be used as a detangler (to detangle the curls). Leave-ins are usually very loose in consistency and similar to water in terms of thickness. They can be used directly on the hair after shampoo for certain curls or used as an extra moisture boost after conditioner but before styling products. Sometimes these products contain sunscreen. Apply by spraying directly to the hair or by hand, and less near the scalp.

Spray Leave-In Conditioners (Cream)

More moisturizing and hydrating than spray leave-in liquid conditioners, cream leave-in conditioners are also heavier, so it's best to spray this product onto your hands first and then apply through the curls with your fingers. This way, you'll ensure even distribution of the product. If sprayed on the hair directly, you may just cover one very small area, and you'll end up using more product than if you apply by hand.

Leave-In Conditioners

Some people who are very curly or super-kinky curly will use a leave-in conditioner on top of conditioner that they have left in. Others may use these products immediately after shampooing or co-washing, relying on the leave-in conditioner for the moisture their curls need, rather than applying then rinsing out a conditioner. It will depend on the moisture level of your curls and how much hydration they're craving; leave-ins can be used as a styling product for extra moisture after you have washed and conditioned your hair. These products come in all sorts of consistencies: creamy, milky colored, clear, loose or thick, or gelatinous. Their purpose is the same as a spray leave-in conditioner, but they can provide more weight to the hair for curlies who want more control, and to keep their curls down and not expanding.

Detangling Sprays

These types of products tend to be lightweight with a little moisturizing base to assist in detangling hair. This step would be the very first thing you would apply to your hair after conditioning. Because of their light weight, detangling sprays can also be used as a refresher to wake up curls for next-day hair.

Deep or Protein Treatments

Deep treatments or masks are used to provide extra moisture to curls, keep hair healthy or repair dry or damaged hair. Most conditioning treatments require heat from a dryer, as the heat intensifies the action of the ingredients in the formula. The warmth opens up the hair cuticle, enabling the treatment to penetrate deeper. Some products, however, don't require heat and work at room temperature. Instructions are on the product label, so follow them. There are conditioning treatments that also come in spray form; don't let the lightweight texture deter you. The molecular properties of a liquid compared to a heavy cream may in some cases work better on your curls, because the liquid can penetrate the cuticle more easily. If you don't have a hooded dryer for a treatment, there are hair bonnets that have a hose that can attach to your hair dryer. Most treatments require you to cover your curls with a plastic cap so you can just apply heat from your hair dryer to create the warmth required. You can put a winter toque or scarf over the plastic cap to seal in the heat while the treatment processes. In the summer (or if you are in a warmer climate), you can sit on your patio in the sun and let that be your heat source. Rinse conditioning treatments clean from the hair; they are not products you leave in. After rinsing, use regular conditioner to seal in the beneficial ingredients of the treatment.

Protein treatments target the cuticle and are designed to repair the inner layer of the hair strand. They do not provide moisture as conditioning/ deep conditioning treatments or masks do. Protein treatments help correct protein deficiencies, whereas conditioning treatments deal with the hydration and moisture level of the hair strand. Protein treatments can come in liquid, spray or cream form. Quinoa, soy, wheat and keratin are but a few protein ingredients to look for. Always read the product label for specific instructions concerning use. Some require heat, for example. Mind the time frames and uses per month, as you can add too much protein to your curls, which will make them dry and brittle.

Leave-In Treatments

These products are specifically labeled as such and are left in the hair. Apply as you would a leave-in conditioner. If the product's consistency is thick, it's probably best to spray the product into your hand and rake through the curls with your fingers to avoid spot spraying and not having the curls covered evenly.

Liquid Gels

Gels can be layered on top of conditioner left in the hair. A gel will give your curls support and memory to hold the curl pattern, and give better next-day curls. The gel acts as a cocoon to protect the curls from the elements, such as the heat and cold from outside. Gels are like glue, in a sense, in that they will hold the cuticles down when they dry, thereby reducing the frizz and flyaway factor that curls are generally known for. Alcohol-free gels are curl-friendly, as they are less drying on the hair strand. If the gel has alcohol in it and you don't use a proper base, such as a leave-in conditioner, it can dry out your curls. Sometimes you have to sacrifice the feel you like for your curls for the control you want over frizz for better next-day curly styling. Some gels will dry hard, others soft; it just depends on the ingredients. Certain gels can leave a softer feeling on the hair when you learn to separate and scrunch your curls when dry.

Spray Gels

Depending on the ingredients, these gels provide either lighter or heavier support for the curls. Spray gels can also create more bounce because their consistency is lighter than a liquid gel's. That said, they tend to spot spray the curls, providing uneven coverage. Spray the gel onto your hand and apply to your hair, or change the spray bottle to one that has a better mist to evenly distribute the product on your curls. These can also make a great alternative to hair spray, especially if you can't find an alcohol-free brand.

Understanding Alcohols

How alcohol-free can it be? There are lots of products with alcohol and some even claim to be alcohol-free. I have suggested alcohol-free products but, in fact, some alcohols are not bad, and some are better than others. It will be a trial-and-error process to see which work best for your curls.

Some alcohols can cause the curls to be dry and really frizzy, while other alcohols can condition the curls. The following alcohols can be more drying: ethanol, SD alcohol, alcohol 40 denat. (denatured alcohol), propanol, propyl alcohol and isopropyl alcohol. These alcohols are "miscible" in water (can mix with water). They evaporate quickly to help hair dry faster, but can result in drying out the curly hair strand and making it frizzy.

The preferred and more conditioning curl-friendly group of alcohol is fatty alcohols. This group includes lanolin, laurel, cetyl, myristyl, stearyl, cetearyl and behenyl alcohol. These alcohols are typically derived from natural sources. The only downside of these alcohols is they can make the hair look greasy when combined with the natural sebum formed on the scalp.

Pick the best curl-friendly ingredient options for your curls to minimize dehydration and frizz. But all in all, alcohol is alcohol, so choose products with alcohol in small percentages (lower on the list of ingredients on the bottle) to minimize the negative and drying effects alcohol can be known for. Usually applying a moisturizing base of a leave-in conditioner will add a protective layer to the cuticle to counter the negative effects of low concentrations of alcohol.

Styling Creams

These products tend to have a richer consistency than a leave-in/leave-on conditioner. Very moisturizing, styling creams are used to hydrate and define curls. Tighter and kinky curl hair types would benefit from this product, because their curls, in most cases, have good memory (retain the curl pattern) but need lots of moisture from a product that is less drying, ingredient-wise. If a styling cream is applied first, a gel can be used on top to lock in the moisturizing benefits. Styling creams tend to add weight to the hair and keep the curls down and from expanding.

Mousses

Packaged in pressurized containers, mousses, like foams, are traditionally lightweight products, but are heavier in consistency. With the advancement of product development, I have seen deep conditioners and leave-in/leave-on conditioners sold in this type of packaging. Styling mousse can be more moisturizing and conditioning for the curls than a foam. The styling results will be similar to what you would achieve using a gel, but without the weight and stickiness associated with the final dry curly style of many gels. Mousses can be used on all curls, but finer curl patterns prefer lightweight products to encourage curls and not weigh them down.

Foams

These usually come in a pump form and act the same way a mousse would, except foams are typically air activated and do not rely on butane to change the liquid to a foam. Some foams can work effectively on all textures but are best for finer-texture curls because foams usually don't weigh curls down. Foams can be designed for use as a treatment, conditioner or styling product. Follow instructions regarding use.

> **Note:** *These next three products come in handy when you learn about styling your curls. A light mist of oil can be used to lubricate the palm of your hand to reduce frizz associated with touching curls when diffusing. Serums and pomades can help break product cast (the firmness left from gel when it's dried). When scrunching the hair to soften the style and break apart curls, a little pomade or serum goes a long way and can also help reduce frizz. That's just a teaser to let you know what's in store in the "Styling Your Curls" chapter!*

Styling Product Silicones & Oils (Not olive, coconut or kitchen-inspired cooking oils)

Intended for adding sheen and for sealing curls, oils should be the last step when used as a styling product. It's the oil that will create a water-repellent layer that will lock in the ingredients of a leave-in/leave-on conditioner. However, oils can dehydrate curls with constant use; over time, they can actually make the hair look dull, so use sparingly, if at all. Clarifying hair every three to four weeks (instructions in the "Washing & Conditioning" chapter) will remove the buildup. Deep condition after clarifying to restore the hair to its proper pH balance. Some oils labeled as "Shine Sprays" are designed to seal moisture in the hair and should be the last styling product applied.

Be mindful of products containing high concentrations of oils unless the formulations make these ingredients water soluble. Silicones are synthetic plastics and not emollients. They coat the hair much like oils, except oils can be removed with a little elbow grease. Silicones remain on the hair and need a special salon service or product designed for clarifying. Most clarifying or chelating shampoos will strip the hair, so it's a vicious cycle to be on. It's best to avoid silicones!

Serums

These products are usually heavier than an oil and are used to seal the ends of hair and control frizz by smoothing down the cuticle. Serums are not really necessary to apply anywhere except the outer layer of curls for that frizz control.

Pomades

Sold in jars, tubs and tubes, pomades add weight (and sometimes shine) to the hair and provide great support for accenting pieces and curls in short haircuts. They are usually oil-based and make hair greasy, so they need to be washed out by clarifying more frequently to reduce the chance of buildup.

Waxes

These styling products are similar to pomades and have similar uses for shorter styles: to accent short cuts and keep hair in place. They can have a semi-matte finish, depending on ingredients.

Hair Putty and Clays

These are sometimes more moisturizing than pomades and waxes, and create more of a matte finish, but they can provide curl control. Hair putty and clays will usually rinse out more easily than waxes and pomades.

Hair Spray

Hair spray can control frizz and flyaways on the hair surface. It's best to find one without alcohol, which is less drying on the curls. If you want to control wavy hair from dropping its curl, hair spray may be the key when applied to dried hair. Be careful not to use hair spray on hair that is tightly pulled back at the hairline, as it will alter the curl pattern and ruin the elasticity of the hair, eventually causing breakage. For special occasions, it's okay to use hair spray to style with. Restore moisture stripped by the hair spray back to your curls the next time you wash your hair, and deep condition really well afterwards to restore the elasticity. Hair spray can be found in aerosol or pump spray. I prefer the pump spray, because it doesn't have the butane needed to propel the spray as the aerosol does and is therefore less drying to curls. You can make your own hair spray by using an alcohol-free gel diluted with a little water (try ¾ ounce gel and ¼ ounce water) put in a little spray bottle and spritz in spots when you do want to control frizz or have a smoother hairstyle.

Sea Salt Sprays

A popular styler for the wavy-curl types, sea salt sprays can be used on wet or dry hair as a styler or even a curl refresher. Typically, these sprays don't provide a lot of hold but are great for a tousled, undone, beachy effect.

Curl Refreshers

These are products sprayed into the hair to revitalize curls. They are light-weight and will reactivate and refresh the styling product you applied the previous day without diluting or dissolving it too much. You'll get better second-day hair if you go a little heavier with your styling product on your wash and style day. You can probably get away with a light mist of water to reactivate the product and refresh your curls. By day three, if you keep spraying water on your curls, you'll dissolve the styling product and may find your hair gets frizzy. This is when a curl refresher comes in handy. Mist some curl refresher on the outer layer, and with the palm of your hand, smooth down the hair to get rid of the frizz; then scrunch the curls and go. Frizz is an indicator of curls looking for moisture. Feed your thirsty curls what they crave. *A three-ounce spray bottle with water and a teaspoon to a tablespoon of conditioner makes a good homemade curl refresher. Shake well before applying a light mist on your hair to reactivate curls and reduce frizz.*

> **Note:** *Use the "plopping" method with a curl refresher to reactivate your curls, as explained in the "Drying Your Curls" chapter.*

What does the phrase "Has good slip" mean to a curly?

Some curlies pick product based on the type of slip it gives to the hair. "Slip" refers to the spreadability of a product on the curls, or the ability of fingers or a comb to pass through the hair after you've applied your product. Some may want a certain texture for their curls and base their choice on the "product slip," how their curls feel once the conditioner or styling product is applied. Some prefer light products, while others heavier. Usually someone with a fine-texture wavy curl will not want to use a heavy product if she wants to maximize her waves, given it will weigh down the hair, preferring instead a light slip. Those with tighter curls, on the other hand, will want the maximum amount of moisture in their hair products to hydrate curls. The tighter the curls, the more moisture they need.

> **Note:** *Don't throw away a product if you feel it is too heavy or sticky. Try diluting a small batch with distilled water or boiled water that has been cooled; don't dilute the whole bottle. Alternatively, this same product may not have worked well on your curls in the summer when you purchased it, but you may find it will work better in the winter because of its formulation. Yes, some products may be seasonal, so learn to read your curls and what they need and when.*

Product Junkie or Jump-Around Curly

Try to stay consistent when trying a new product. Don't be so quick to jump from product to product. Give the new one a few good tries before calling it quits. Seventy-five percent of the time it's the method of application that is at fault, not the product. So do make sure you are applying products as instructed in the "Styling Your Curls" chapter—coming up shortly. Each little step has a purpose in creating the desired end result: a great finished style.

Eliminate Product Buildup

If over time you feel your products (the ones you love so much for your hair) are not working for you, try the clarifying method to start with a clean curly slate. A gentle and effective way to remove product buildup is to use baking soda and sulfate-free shampoo; instructions are found in the "Washing & Conditioning" chapter. If you're concerned about how the clarifying will affect your processed hair color or highlights, do a strand test. I have yet to see any negative effects on processed hair that has been clarified with baking soda and sulfate-free shampoo.

So, curlies, it will be trial and error to find what works and doesn't work for your hair, product-wise. The "Styling Your Curls" chapter will show you how to apply your products properly, which is crucial to making them work effectively for you.

Oils: When to use them and how.

If you find you need to use oils for a dry scalp, the best to use are the oils your scalp naturally produces. Upon going into the shower, use warm water to soften the oils on the scalp, then use your fingertips in a circular motion to massage the natural oils into your scalp and down the hair strands as a pre-cleansing step. Don't use cold or cooler water, as it will not soften the natural scalp oils, but harden them. Think of how a greasy pan reacts when you pour cold water into it to clean instead of warmer water. However, if you feel your scalp needs more oil than what is being produced naturally, consider jojoba oil; jojoba is similar in consistency to the sebum our scalps naturally create. Simply coat your fingertips with a little jojoba oil and massage into your scalp, working on small sections at a time. Massaging the scalp is beneficial, as it clears the oils blocking the cuticles and stimulates the glands, which is great for healthy hair and hair growth. A healthy scalp means healthier hair.

Never use oils straight from the bottle on your hair as a treatment. Oils block the oxygen your hair and scalp need to breathe. Despite what you might think, oils do not moisturize the hair: a good conditioner will moisturize your hair. You can use a little oil as a final step after applying styling product, or after hair is styled and dried to seal in the styling product's moisturizing ingredients. But understand that once you have sealed your hair with any type of oil, no other product you use on top will be able to penetrate the hair shaft. This means you won't be able to refresh your curls the next day with a curl refresher or a light misting of water. You will just end up a curly mess. What happens if you spray water on a greasy pan? It does nothing. The water just sits on top of the oil. Also, be mindful of using products with a high concentration of oil in their ingredients.

Using oil over and over on your hair will lead to your curls becoming brittle—in some cases, excessive use can even cause hair to become more fragile and cause breakage. Over time, oil will create a matte-looking hazy appearance to the surface of your hair. Using oil straight from the bottle on the hair will also cause the negative effects you are trying to avoid, such as frizz and dryness.

Keep in mind there are different kinds and qualities of oil. Most oils contain fillers and other products that do more harm than good to your curly strands. If you feel you need to use oil, using a little bit of 100 percent pure argan oil will be more effective when applied on top of a leave-in conditioner to the ends of your hair instead of the olive oil you use for cooking. Olive oil, even in its purest form, is too heavy for the hair. Macadamia nut oil is a good alternative, as it is very light and easily absorbed into the scalp. If an oil feels light and slips well on your fingers, it will be far more beneficial than a heavy-feeling oil.

The straighter and thicker the hair strands, the tighter the cuticles are and therefore the harder it is for oils to penetrate and cause as many negative effects (as noted above) as it would for a curlier hair type (i.e., 3 to 4 patterns). The curlier the hair as we move from 1 to 4 on the curl pattern chart, the more dehydrating oils are on that hair. Those in the kinky curly 4 pattern seem to be the curlies falling into overuse of oil as a remedy for dry curls. What I want you kinky curly curls to know is sometimes your hair texture will never look shiny or glossy. When you add oil to make it look shiny, you are actually drying out your hair. Castor oils and concoctions are better left aside. Yes, that's correct. I'm telling you the castor oil suggested for you to use for generations back is not a remedy for dry curls. Washing less and conditioning more is the best remedy for dry curls. Overuse with the oil will leave your hair a tangled mess when you wash, as I'm sure you're finding. Being a curl type that is the most fragile because of the kinks and coils (the more bends in the hair, the more fragile your curls are), you may experience breakage and excessive shedding, and therefore feel your curls are never growing! These negative side effects of using oils are only enhanced by using shampoo in an attempt to remove the oil you have put on your curls to make them feel soft and shiny. The excessive washing of your curls makes them super-dry, so you start over again layering oils in an attempt to hydrate and create shine. It's a vicious curly cycle. To make matters worse, if you use polyester scarves, bonnets and wraps to protect your curls when you have oil on your hair, you are doubling the suffocating effects of the oil, as your scalp cannot breathe. What happens when you put oil in a pan and heat it? It cooks and fries your food. Locking all the heat in your scalp and hair under the bonnet has the same effect: you're cooking your curls. Time to stop oil frying your curls.

Remedy for Oil Junkies: Clarifying

Don't rush to the beauty supply shop or drugstore looking for another product to add to your collection. You don't need to buy a clarifying or chelating shampoo to remove the oil and buildup. Chances are these products will have sulfates or other ingredients that will be harsh on your curls. The solution can be found right in your kitchen cupboard. Use baking soda and sulfate-free shampoo to clarify and remove buildup from your curls. This is explained in Chapter 4, "Washing & Conditioning."

Clarifying is only to be done once a month to remove the oil. If you're a kinky curly and have done the clarifying to give your hair a fresh start, feel free to wet down your hair as much as you want thereafter, but do not shampoo—just co-wash with your conditioner. Wash your curls with conditioner, wet down with conditioner, and condition with conditioner. CONDITION. CONDITION. CONDITION. That's your BFF, my curly friend, until you restore the moisture to your curls caused by the dehydrating and negative effects of oil use.

Layering Styling Products

Do you have a cupboard full of products as you try this and that, but find that your curly style is just not working? This chapter will help you understand how to *layer* your styling products properly to get better results. The "Styling Your Curls" chapter will show you *how* to apply these products. Some products are designed to be put on the hair first for optimal results. Usually there are instructions on the label. Others can be used at more than one stage when styling. An example would be a conditioning spray or detangler that says you apply to freshly washed wet curls or used on dry hair to refresh your curls. Another example is a leave-in conditioner, a product, you learned earlier, that is left in the hair. The leave-in is to be applied to your curls first, before adding any other products. The exception would be if you're using a detangling spray, which would instead be the first product. Sectioning the hair and layering the products properly will give you a better finished curly style and better frizz control—two things all curlies strive for.

Here's the order of applying your styling products for the best results, whether you use one styling product or are layering them.

1. Detangling spray or conditioning serum
2. Leave-in conditioner (can be a foam, styling cream or lotion)
3. Gel (liquid or spray)
4. Mousse or styling foam
5. Pomade
6. Hair spray

7. Light layer of oil or shine spray. Any product that is oil based I would use last in order to seal in the other products that may have nourishing ingredients for curls, such as proteins.
8. Curl refresher

Check the label for the product's intended use. The above list is just a sampling of the product categories, as styling products can come in different forms. For example, a foam can be a conditioning foam to be used as the second product you would apply, or a styling and volumizing foam to be the fourth product you would apply.

I consider a leave-in conditioner a styling product. One mistake some lazy curlies make when applying their products is to put all the styling products together in their hands all at once (called a cocktail) and apply all over. Without sectioning the hair or being mindful to apply the products in layers, you are going to get uneven results and the products will not deliver the desired results. Also, if you use a leave-in with proteins, this key ingredient won't get properly sealed into your curls if not applied first. You dilute the effectiveness of each product when you mix them together this way. A curly who has really dry hair will need a leave-in conditioner applied in lotion or spray form to help with curl hydration before applying anything else. That's not to say that sometimes two products in the same category can't be mixed together to give you a great curly style, but usually it's best to apply in categories as above when using more than one.

Some curlies are content using a leave-in conditioner (or conditioner left in their hair) as their styling product. Most good-quality leave-ins will have some form of protein that feeds—and in some cases, adds thickness to—the hair strand, providing much-needed moisture to reduce frizz.

If you are a curly who likes gel, that product would be the next one you would use on your curls. It's best to layer gel on top of the leave-in, or any conditioner you have left in your hair, especially if there are oils or alcohol in the gel. The conditioner will buffer the curls from the drying effects of the gel and oil penetration. If gel is the only product you are using as a styling product, it would be applied (according to recommendations in the

"Styling Your Curls" chapter) right after lightly removing some moisture from your curls. Gel is a great product to surround, or cocoon, the cuticle with a protective layer to combat frizz during high humidity; it can also protect curls from extreme heat from hair dryers. *Alcohol-free gel is best, as it's less drying and damaging to the curly hair strand.*

The next product layer you would apply is a styling foam or mousse. Most foams do not provide enough support for a good curly style, or curl encouragement and memory for next-day curls. For best next-day curls, you would need another product to partner with it for curl retention. Foams and mousses pair nicely when applied on top of a leave-in conditioner. Foams are lightweight and should be the last product you apply to your curls, unless you're using hair spray or oils as a finisher.

Once curls are dried, the next product would be a pomade. If using, take an appropriate amount for your curls' length and thickness. I have short medium-textured curls and I use a double pea-sized amount. Rub the pomade in your hands so you have a light layer of product evenly coated on your fingers and palms. Take your hair in a ponytail atop your head (no matter how short your hair) and scrunch down the hair shaft from root to ponytail end to break the product cast (the thin layer left on hair from the leave-in conditioner, gel, mousse, etc.) for your finished style.

Next comes hair spray. My wavy curls love this product for frizzy flyaway control. The challenge is to find a hair spray that is alcohol-free. A spray bottle or pump is better than an aerosol, as butane in the aerosol can be drying. Hair spray is usually applied after you have broken the product cast and/or shuffled your hair to loosen the curl (you'll learn about this in "Styling Your Curls") or sprayed on your hair without loosening the curl for a more put-together curly look. Spray bottle applicators sometimes apply too much concentration of hair spray in one area, so if using a pump or spray bottle, you can also apply the hair spray to your palm and graze the product by hand down the curly strand to apply a light, even coat to the outside layer.

After hair spray comes the oils. This curly stylist suggests you use a light hand (so very little of this product) if using. A light layer of oil can be applied on wet curls (after your leave-in conditioner, or gels or mousses). Most commonly, however, oils are applied when curls are dry to lock in the moisture benefits from the other products (especially a good leave-in product or conditioner). Go light with this oil step, as you don't want to suffocate and weigh down the curls.

Finally are the curl refreshers, to be used between wash days, to wake up curls after getting out of bed or for controlling frizz throughout the day. The product works well to reactivate your previously applied styling products on wash day. Curl refreshers won't be effective if used over oils (that are not water soluble), though, given oils repel water and most refreshers will have water as their main ingredient.

Make Your Own Curl Refresher

You can make your own refresher by mixing your favorite curly styling products in a spray bottle, following one of these three options:

- 1 part gel, 1 part conditioner and 4 parts water
- 1 part leave-in conditioner and ¾ part water (for 3 and 4 curl patterns)
- 3 ounces of distilled water and one teaspoon to one tablespoon of conditioner for finer hair textures (for a light curl refresher)

Use bottled or boiled and cooled water for your curl refreshers. Some curlies like aloe vera juice as a curl refresher, but it can be a tad sticky. You can incorporate aloe vera juice into any of the above mixtures. You'll have to experiment to see what proportion will work best when making your curl refresher and adjust your recipe accordingly.

Make small two- to three-ounce batches so your spray is always fresh. Also, making smaller batches leaves room to adjust and add more water if needed to dilute a curl refresher you have mixed that may be too heavy for your curls. Store in the fridge, because a cool mist works best on some curls.

Use a spray bottle that mists the product on your curls, rather than shoots a stream at one curl. A spray bottle that gently mists the curls is a must-have for a curl refresher. Once applied, graze your palms down along the curls to smooth the surface, then gently scrunch the curls in your hands to reactivate. Let your curls be until dry—too much touching could cause excessive frizz.

> **Note:** *Remember, frizz is simply curls looking for moisture. A spray bottle of water with a little conditioner would be an easy DIY solution to combat frizz. I always style my hair on wash day with a little more styling product so that my curl refresher (water and conditioner) can be used for at least three days without diluting my styling-product base too much before I have to wash and style my hair again.*

Chapter 6

To Comb
or Not to Comb?

That is the curly question. Cute play with words on a sensitive curly matter. Most curlies I meet will admit to using a comb when they wash their hair, as they find they just can't detangle their curls properly by fingers alone. And I have converted many a curly in my studio by using a comb when styling their curly locks; they love the results so much, they end up implementing this method to get the best curly results at home. With my clients, I do a comparison test so they can see how different the curls feel when applying product by fingers compared to using a comb. In some cases, depending on curl pattern or length of hair, I choose a brush for applying product.

Using either a comb or brush is a frizz-busting product application method that also saves time. Some clients at the beginning of their curl journey start by styling their hair using the comb method until their curls' moisture level has been restored, thanks to the changes in their curly hair routines.

Once their hair has gone into full curl recovery (sometimes it takes weeks or months), the clients will change to applying product by fingers. If you're opposed to using a comb or brush on your curls and prefer to use your fingers, no worries—there is still a lot you can pick up here even if you choose not to incorporate this chapter into your routine. In the "Styling Your Curls" chapter, you'll learn more about how to use your fingers to apply product correctly, if that's your preference.

Combs have a bad reputation when it comes to some curly methods. But I find them a very effective way to move a client along in her curl journey. They can help to hydrate the hair when applying conditioner and styling product, resulting in a great finished curly style with reduced frizz. Why? Think of it this way: Using five fingers to apply product down each curly strand that has thousands of small cuticle layers compared to using a medium-spaced tooth comb running down each strand. It's as though the comb has 20 little fingers forcing the product right into each crevice (cuticle). If you're trying to control small raised portions down the hair strand such as the cuticle, it makes sense to use a smaller tool such as a comb to create a smooth surface, instead of hands and fingers running through the layers, which in effect are only smoothing a small percentage of the cuticle. Big fingers to a thin strand—use a comb, and you are using something relatively closer in proportion to the thing you are trying to control: the cuticle, and frizz by association. Which one do you think will help the product coat the curls better? Hands down, the comb wins.

And no, combs and brushes do not ruin the curl pattern. Nor will using a comb to apply styling product make your hair and curls look stringy. You can discount any other negative comments out there concerning using a comb or brush on curly hair. As long as there is plenty of moisture (water) left in your curls and the curls are conditioned well, both methods work perfectly. Using a comb the correct way can give your curls the TLC, "Tender Love & Conditioner," they need! Combs, and in some cases brushes, push conditioner into each little crevice and cuticle, providing a smoothness to the surface that can't be achieved on dehydrated hair with finger application alone. They are master curly hair tools and frizz

busters when applying products to the outer layer of curls, the "halo," where curls are most prone to frizz.

Combing your curls is an effective method worth incorporating into your routine, but you have to use the comb correctly. It's important that your hair is properly hydrated (see Moisture Level Test, p. 68 in the "Styling Your Curls" chapter) and conditioned when using a comb for the styling portion of your routine. When you apply conditioner (as you learned in the "Washing & Conditioning" chapter), it is important to let it sit on the hair to process and penetrate the cuticle for a few minutes. After the processing time, you could use a wide-tooth comb or Pik to detangle the hair. Curls must be detangled for the most part with a wide-tooth comb, rake or Pik before you move to a comb that has the teeth spaced closer together. They also need to be well hydrated so the hair will stretch and release knots without breaking from excessive tugging.

If your curls are damaged and hair is in a fragile state, then I do not recommend combs or brushes, especially on dry curls, as the hair may break. When hair is wet, it has a little more stretch, so if you wish to comb, that would be the time. Healthy, hydrated and properly conditioned hair can stretch up to two times its length and bounce back without breaking. You can test your curls according to the instructions in the "Curl Pattern & Elasticity" chapter.

The rule of thumb for 2 and 3 curl patterns is to comb your hair from roots to ends. When you come upon a knot or a tangle, remove the comb and begin detangling curls from the ends up to where the knot is in small sections half the width of your comb, or approximately two-inch sections across. You will lose less hair this way and get rid of the knot. Most knots are caused by a few strands of naturally shed hair tangling with the curls, curls matted from sleeping routine or poor-quality products being used. Washing your curls too often is also a big culprit for creating masses of knots and matted hair, as it causes the cuticles to raise excessively; the raised dry cuticle appearing as frizz is attaching to every other curly frizz on the other strands. Control the frizz by hydrating your hair with good conditioner and you'll decrease the knots and matting. As you change your routines according to the lessons learned in *The ABCs*, the knots and matting of curls will lessen over time. You'll be able to remove the knots or untangle your hair more effectively without pulling out unshed hair from the roots that is caught in the knot. One loose shedding hair can grab 10 or more healthy unshed strands, *so take your time.* If a knot is really hard to detangle, apply conditioner and allow it to remain on the hair a few minutes, then add a few trickles of water and use your fingers to separate the knot. Then use a really wide-tooth comb before changing to a regular detangling comb once the knot has been removed.

> ***Note:*** *The "Styling Your Curls" chapter (Choices for Application) will explain using the comb as your styling product application tool.*

For tighter and kinkier hair patterns (3s and 4s), first apply a lot of conditioner to hydrate your curls, then use your fingers to detangle very knotted hair followed by a wide-tooth comb to further detangle. Finish detangling with a paddle brush (preferably with soft bristles), brushing out small sections of hair by working in a downward motion from **ends to roots of each section**. Finally, smooth conditioner through from **roots to ends.**

What types of combs and brushes are for curls and what do they do?

Here is a breakdown of the types of combs and brushes relevant to curly hair and curly hair styling.

Rake Combs with or without handles are great for detangling, as they mimic finger detangling. The wide teeth of this style comb are spaced far apart, providing minimal pulling on the hair and providing a good way to getting rid of larger knots and tangles. Don't worry if your hair is knotty as you start your curl journey. It takes some time to get your curls rehydrated and to a better state. The more dehydrated the hair, the more frizz and the more tangles.

Detangling Combs are very sturdy, with thicker teeth to detangle hair gently. Most have a handle and come in different sizes and different thicknesses of teeth; thicker comb teeth are more suitable for thick and coarse curl types. These combs are also good for combing through your conditioner.

Double Detangling Combs are also sturdy, and are especially good for those with really coarse hair, but will work on finer hair textures, as well. The combs have double rows of teeth either close together, with the rows almost touching, or spaced farther apart. These combs whiz through knotty, tangled hair much more effectively than single-tooth combs because of the way the teeth overlap and effectively distribute conditioner easily through curls.

Grooming Combs, also referred to as dressing or pocket combs, are suggested for coarse hair in the 3 to 4 curl pattern categories, as they have wider-spaced teeth. Sometimes there are two different teeth spacings on the comb. One end has finer teeth spaced closely together, while the other end has thicker teeth spaced farther apart. These combs are excellent for applying your styling product.

Styling, or Cutting, Combs are for fine hair in the 1 to 2 curl pattern categories. As above, some combs will have two different spacings and thicknesses of teeth on one comb. Cutting combs have slightly angled teeth and are used by hairstylists for cutting hair, but for our purpose, this comb makes a great tool for applying styling product.

Tail Combs are also for finer hair. This type of comb is a great way to lift hair that's stuck to your scalp after applying your styling product. You can use the tail end of the comb not only to lift the hair, but also to correct your part line. It's a handy multi-function styling tool. Tail combs are not airplane-friendly, however, because of their pointy ends, so make sure, if you do start to love your tail comb as much as I love mine, to pack it with your luggage, or the comb will more than likely be confiscated through airport security if packed in your carry-on bag.

Paddle, or Wet, Brushes are an effective way to apply conditioner or styling product and can help elongate 3 to 4 pattern curls. The paddle brush generally has very fine, soft nylon bristles (some paddle brushes have small plastic balls at the tip of the bristles to protect the scalp from being scratched) and is great to use on the scalp to stimulate the sebaceous glands to encourage the production of natural oils. Curls in the 3 to 4 categories tend to be on the drier side, and there is nothing better for your hair than for your natural hair oils to be distributed through your curls. It's best to detangle your hair first with a wide-tooth comb and then work from the mid-shaft down the curly strand, then slowly back up to the root with each stroke of the brush. Alternatively, you can start from the ends of your curls and move upwards a couple of inches at a time if you have very tight kinky curls. These brushes will also work well on 1 to 2 curl patterns and are ideal for to distributing conditioner and applying styling product.

Denman Brushes have rubber bristles and can work the same way as paddle brushes work, except the bristles are a lot firmer. Follow the same method as you would for the paddle brush when using the Denman brush. I personally think the paddle brush will be a more effective way to gently spread product through your curls. Do test for yourself.

Piks at one time were used exclusively in Afro textures to make the hair more voluminous. They are an effective way to get oxygen to the scalp where denser hair tends to clump together and cause the scalp to suffocate. Piks are not only great for detangling curls after applying conditioner, but also for holding up finer hair so your curls are out of the shower stream when conditioning. The downside to some Piks, though, is that the material used to make them is very rigid, and the tips of the Pik can scratch the scalp, so use care when using a firm plastic Pik close to your scalp.

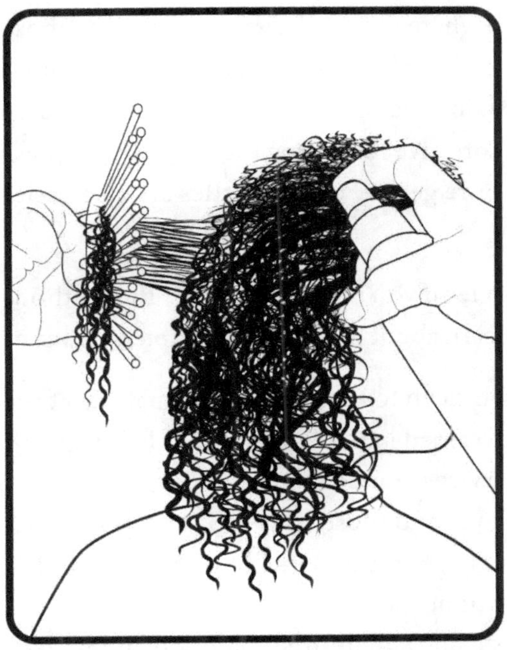

Use a Pik to apply spray styling products.

Combs and Piks make wonderful styling product assistants when using products that dispense from a spray or pump bottle. Hold your hair out from the scalp when combing from root to end, then mist the product (e.g., leave-in conditioner or spray gel) on section by section. This way, the product will be evenly distributed, rather than just hitting the top layer of curls.

There are numerous styles of combs and brushes available for detangling hair and applying styling product, so do your research. And don't go cheap on curly hair tools! If you were a flat-iron junkie before and invested $150 on a good flat iron, $20 to $40 for a good comb or brush will be a worthwhile investment. Take care of the tools: keeping them clean will prolong their lifespan.

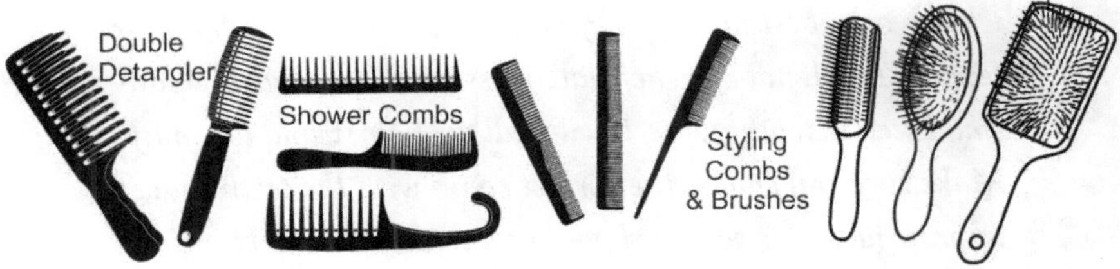

I recommend and prefer handmade combs from various parts of the world. They range from $15 to $30. Handmade combs are smooth with a hand-polished finish and no seams to cause breakage or stress on the hair. The seams on mass-produced, machine-made combs can have really sharp edges between each tooth where the comb sits in the mould. Those sharp edges can cut into and break curls. I also prefer medium-textured nylon bristles on a paddle brush instead of natural bristles, because they are soft and flexible and have more give for styling the curls when applying product, so are therefore more gentle; nylon bristles are also easier to clean.

Don't get discouraged with tangles if you're a curl newbie. The methods you've learned about (and will learn about in upcoming chapters), such as

- protecting hair when you sleep to keep curls from matting at the nape of your neck (as explained in the "Sleeping Curly" chapter);
- altering the chemical services you do to your curls;
- not using poor-quality dyes and those with PPD and ammonia;
- not using foil highlights (as explained in Chapter 11, "Color & Highlights"); and, most importantly,
- better washing routines using sulfate-free shampoo and hydrating conditioners

will all aid in decreasing the tangles you've experienced and help you in your curl journey. Using the proper combs and brushes is simply another method to consider implementing to better hydrate your curls when conditioning and assist when applying styling products.

> **Note:** *Test your curls using different combs and brushes to see what works best for you. If you use too fine a comb for your texture, it will not be beneficial unless you work through really small sections; otherwise, it will pull the hair strand too much. Make sure you choose the correct comb with the teeth spaced appropriately for your curl pattern and the size of sections you plan to work through. Always make sure to use a wide-tooth comb or rake comb first to do a pre-detangling of the curls. You can use the finer-toothed comb after the main detangling is done.*

You may even choose to detangle with just a wide-tooth comb and save the detailing comb of your choice for the outer layer as a frizz buster.

The top layer of curls (your halo, curly angel) are more prone to frizz and dryness because that area is exposed to the elements. Your curls underneath the top layers tend to be smoother, in general. Using the comb method specifically on the top layer will smooth down that halo, force the moisturizing benefits of your leave-in conditioner into each layer and provide much-needed hydration to that protective layer. You will learn more about all this in the following chapter, "Styling Your Curls." It's the longest chapter in *The ABCs*, so get ready for me to totally rock your curly world with what comes next!

Chapter 7

Styling Your Curls

Styling curls. Huge chapter, right? You must be thinking, "If I have to read 13 sections on styling, how long will it take me to style my curls?" Exhale, curly, don't despair! What follows is really quick and easy. My curly clients don't have a lot of time to spend on their curls. With today's busy lifestyles, most of us don't have a lot of time for our hair, so less time spent styling our hair means more time to juggle life! But less time does not mean compromising. It's all about streamlining the styling routine and maximizing the curly style—putting all the steps of this puzzle together in the ABCs so you get the great curly style you've envisioned.

Okay, so seriously, back to this 13-section chapter. It's not as bad as it looks. For example, if you're a medium-texture curly with medium-length hair (curls fall at the shoulder), once you've learned the styling routine, implementing it should take you roughly two to three minutes (not including, obviously, drying time). Hopefully that example makes you feel better about the time involved in styling. Keep in mind that styling routines and time will, of course, depend on the length and thickness of your curls. If you have thick, super-kinky hair, it goes without saying you'll need more time.

When a new curly client books a curl coaching session at Curly Girls Studio, the session lasts at least two hours. The styling portion takes the longest amount of time. This "Styling Your Curls" chapter contains a lot of info for your curls. But keep in mind, this book is for all curl patterns, so I have included various methods incorporating different techniques for using and applying products. Each method meets a different need for your curls and will contribute to the finished style in a different way. For example, finger raking is an effective method for applying product, but if your hair is really dehydrated, you may wish to implement the comb or brush method, as it will save time and effort when applying the product, and provide a better final curl style result.

The most important thing to keep in mind is that each method will have the same curly hair foundation: super-wet, well-hydrated (conditioned) curls. Remember this: *If your curls look frizzy when wet, your curls will be even more frizzy when dry.* You have to watch for this as you're styling your hair and make sure to take the necessary steps to remedy this when the curls are wet, or you'll end up with a less than satisfactory finished curly style. If you're new to being curly, understand that it will take time for your curls to overcome frizziness from your previous not-so-curl-friendly routines. Just be patient, put in the time and effort in the beginning and it will get easier every time you style your curls, and the frizz will slowly become under control.

In this chapter you will learn:

1. MOST IMPORTANT: How much water (moisture) needs to be left in your curls as a base before applying styling product.
2. How to do the "cuticle check" to ensure a smooth, curly finish.
3. How to apply styling product.
4. How to section, style and add volume to your curl—plus so much more!

When I began working on this chapter, I quickly realized that it is totally different teaching someone with a specific curl pattern how to do a new routine face to face. The challenge was finding how to build a chapter to help all the different curlies grasp the concepts and implement a new curly styling lifestyle as simply as possible. Not so simple! I have tried to take into consideration as many variables as I could, because providing you with such a highly detailed chapter will help ensure you understand the styling steps necessary to be successful at styling your curls, just as if we were face to face in the studio.

If you are new to implementing curly routines, don't be discouraged if your curls still go frizzy, or your curls drop and can't hold their shape after following all the ABCs. Dehydrated curls will take awhile to recover from your old hair routines. Depending on your curly "hairstory" (history of curl abuse) and how bad the damage is to your curl pattern, it may take your hair weeks, months or even longer to reach its true curly potential.

Once you begin to restore moisture to your hair (not stripping it with sulfates in shampoo), apply conditioner properly and implement the other steps you will learn here, your curls will come along in no time. The elasticity will eventually return to your curls. (Remember the hair's ability to hold a curl is primarily based on the elasticity?) Most curlies see a drastic improvement with the first session at the studio, and their curls continue to improve over the following weeks once they implement the new curl-friendly routines. With patience, and the time you invest learning the lessons in *The ABCs*, you will get your curls to where they are meant to be. Little by little you will get the hang of your new curly routine and be on your way to a great curly lifestyle!

Step one in achieving great curly results is leaving the right amount of water in your curls before applying styling product. If you don't do this first step properly, your curly style will be an F. My curly clients always pass with A+ in curly styling when getting this step down! Read the next section carefully and keep these formulas in mind as you move throughout the styling sections.

Removing Too Much Moisture + Raised Cuticles + Products Not Hydrating Enough + Incorrect Methods = Frizzy Hot Mess

Proper Moisture Balance + Smooth Cuticles + Products
Layered Properly + Solid Curly Methods = Amazing
Controlled Curls + Curl Retention + Less Frizz

Moisture Level Test: For perfectly styled curls

In cosmetology, we learned that to get smooth results with our wet sets, perms, barrel curls, roller sets or finger wave, we must keep hair super-wet as we sectioned the hair to achieve an A+ in our finished style. Mrs. Armstrong would be testing and checking and reminding us of this as we styled our mannequins. We kept our spray bottles handy to make sure the hair also remained super-wet (not just damp) throughout the whole styling process, spraying water on each section if it became too dry as we moved from section to section. Curls need the right amount of moisture to produce a great finished curly style. If you're one who leaves water in, I'm sure it's still nowhere near the amount I leave in for styling curls! Every curly client I meet always comments on how much water I have left in the hair when styling. Once I have finished styling the curls and the hair is dried, my curly client is a convert for keeping the curls super-wet when applying styling products. *One of the keys to a successful curly style is to begin with super-wet curls.*

When curls are not hydrated enough, styling products:

- can't penetrate the cuticle properly for frizz control
- just sit on top of the curly strand and are ineffective
- don't spread properly

Why is it beneficial to the finished style to have curls this wet?

First, the cuticle is in a totally different position when hair is completely wet from when it's dry. When hair dries, the cuticles slowly raise up if dehydrated. The goal is to make sure we have the cuticles saturated and lying down (as when hair is wet) when applying the styling product to ensure the product is effectively covering the whole hair strand and penetrating each cuticle layer down that hair strand. This way, as the curls dry, there is styling product on top of and thoroughly saturating each little cuticle to act as a glue to keep them down when external forces, such as the elements (hot and cold weather, humidity and dew factor), attach themselves or try to penetrate the cuticle to try to make that cuticle rise up—which will make hair look frizzy.

Starting your styling with that extra moisture required for a better curly style may result in longer drying times for your curls. You will figure out when the best time of the day is to wash and style your curls (to allow your curls to dry in your preferred method) and where the best place is to style your curls; it's a messy job, for example, if you have super-long or thick hair dripping water everywhere. Some curlies will do their styling product application in the shower to keep the moisture level optimal without worrying about having water all over the place. Just monitor your hair's moisture level as you apply your styling product and work quickly while the curls have that proper moisture level. Always keep a spray bottle handy to add more water if needed as you work on each section to keep the cuticles saturated.

After you cleanse your hair and prepare for styling your curls, **you should not:**

- wrap your hair in any towel
- put your hair in a turban
- rub your curls aggressively with your hands or towel to remove moisture

Doing any of the above actions will remove too much moisture, and rubbing the curls just creates raised cuticles, resulting in frizz. Removing excess moisture should be done gently. Squeezing the excess moisture out with a microfiber towel, T-shirt or even a paper towel similar to the ones found at the gym (the brown recycled eco-friendly type).

What is the perfect moisture level for any styling product application?

Hair should be hydrated and feel slippery like seaweed before applying styling product (or your leave-in conditioner). When you gather a handful of curls, they should make a healthy squish sound (the "scrunch test") before you apply your styling product. If your curls don't feel this way or make this sound, you are not using the right conditioner, not applying the conditioner correctly or not leaving enough moisture in your curls, or possibly a combination of the three. **To test the moisture level, scrunch a handful of curls from the ends up to your scalp. If your hair is making an audible squish sound when you gently squeeze that handful of curls—and water is not dripping in excess through your fingers as you do so—you have the perfect moisture level.** Again, it's important to keep a spray bottle handy and spray water as needed during the styling product application to maintain that moisture level. It's not unusual if you need to add water right after washing your hair; some curls dry really quickly or let go of water faster than others.

After I wash/cleanse and condition my clients' hair, I gather the hair from the ends and squeeze out the excess water while scrunching to the roots using a microfiber towel. I then start sectioning and applying styling products. If you find a lot of water is still dripping through your fingers after squeezing with the microfiber towel, repeat the process (gathering hair from ends and scrunching to the roots with the microfiber towel) a second time. Do your scrunch test with your bare hands again to make sure your hair is still making the proper sound and still feels very wet without dripping excessively through your fingers. For very dehydrated curls, I don't remove any moisture at all and, in fact, have to spray more water on after sectioning the hair to make the surface receptive to the styling product.

What's the best thing to use to remove moisture from our hair?

It's best to use either a cotton T-shirt or a microfiber towel to remove excess moisture; when scrunching the hair, you should always use either one of those. You should never take a towel and rub your scalp or rub it on your curls down the hair strand. You want to keep the moisture level optimal for frizz control. You just want to remove any excessive dripping water, and do it gently.

Note: *Do not use a cotton towel, as it will pull too much moisture from the curls. There are looped rough hooks on the towel surface that will attach to the cuticles and cause curls to frizz. Microfiber towels have a smoother surface and are made of a synthetic fiber that gently removes excess moisture when used as described above. Because microfiber has a smoother surface than cotton, there isn't anything for the curly cuticle to hook onto when you're gently removing moisture. As a result, using microfiber towels to remove moisture will reduce frizz. Whether you use a loop-style microfiber towel, which feels plush like a towel, or a chamois-style towel (like ones used to dry windows at the car wash), either will remove moisture better than a cotton towel, and neither will cause excessive frizz. Using a lightweight cotton T-shirt to remove moisture is also preferable to a cotton towel. Because a T-shirt's surface is smooth, it will gently remove extra moisture without causing curls to frizz.*

Curly Tip

When you're applying styling product to each section of hair, test to make sure the moisture level is correct and either remove extra moisture or apply more moisture with a spray bottle of water as you go through the sections as needed. In most cases, you'll be adding, not removing, moisture. If hair is fine or medium texture, just use water from a spray bottle. If hair is coarse, porous and a drier curl pattern, keep handy a spray bottle filled with one tablespoon or more of conditioner and four to six ounces of water to add extra moisture as a good hydrating base for your styling product. If you find you need more moisture in your conditioner mixture, adjust the ratio of water to conditioner accordingly.

Providing a good moisturized base will produce a rocking curly style result. Not doing so will have you sporting a less than optimal curly style, and you won't get the best second-day curls either! Get this step down well, and the rest of the styling steps will easily fall into place.

How Much Product to Use

Some people want great curl texture, definition, bounce and hydration, but don't want to use product. Well, this is not going to happen. You can't achieve all those goals with reasonable expectations without using the products and proper application methods. Others don't like the feel of product on their hair, yet want better next-day curls. Sometimes you have to sacrifice feel for look and longevity of the curly style. I prefer to have my hair last three days. I'll use a little more styling product on my co-wash/styling day to get the time I want out of my curls. In effect, this saves me one wash and style per week.

You will have to let the thickness and texture of your hair be your guide as to how much product to use. Some products' ability to spread on the surface of the hair is better than others, in that a little product with *good slip* goes a long way. "Slip" refers to a product's ability to spread and glide on the curls. Each curl on your head is different, and styling product combinations are endless. Keep in mind, if you are using more than one product to style your curls, you can use less of each product. You have to figure out what styling products work best for your curls. There is no hard and fast rule here. It will be a matter of trial and error for you to figure out. In the following tip, I have set out a product estimate usage guideline.

The key to being successful with styling products and proportion is to get to know your curls and what they need. If they need moisture to feel hydrated, test and see if leaving some of your conditioner in is providing enough moisture to your curls to be a base layer before applying your styling product. Or consider using a true leave-in conditioner or even a product such as a styling cream to provide moisture. Don't be afraid of gels; just try to find alcohol-free products. Using gels can really enhance the definition of your curl pattern and buffer the curls against the dryness of the sun's heat and harshness of the cold, especially when applied on top of a moisturizing base, such as a leave-in conditioner. If a product is not working, change it up or add a layer of another product as a base, or perhaps a product on top to seal like a gel. Don't keep using the same products over and over expecting different results. In most cases, just as curls are complex, you may find it hard to be a "one-product curly" to get the results you want for your curly style. Throw in the complexity of external forces such as humidity, dew points, seasons and climates, and how these factors affect how styling products work on your curls, and you'll understand why it may take time to see what works best for your curls and when to use which one.

Curly Tip

A general guideline for how much styling product to use on a short curly or pixie cut with fine to medium texture is to use about a silver dollar amount of styling product for the whole head of curls. However, a person with really thick hair would use that silver dollar amount in just one "section." Know that you can have the best styling products at your disposal, but if you don't know how to apply them properly, it won't make a difference what you use. You'll learn about sections and how to apply your products in this chapter to maximize your curly style.

Layering Your Products

We covered some of this info in the "Product Knowledge" chapter, but again, if you are using multiple products for your styling, you have to layer them properly. Do not combine all of the products in your hand (called a cocktail), especially if they are marked for specific needs. That doesn't mean you can never mix products together, but detangling products, and leave-on and leave-in conditioners should always be applied alone to provide the base your curls need for hydration—not "cocktailed" with other products that are used for curl encouragement and sealing in moisture, such as gels.

The order of product application is as follows:

- Detangling spray (cream or lotion) or conditioning serum
- Leave-in/leave-on conditioner
- Gel or styling cream or lotion
- Foam or mousse
- Pomade or hair putty or paste
- Spray oil or hair spray

Use a light hand with oil on curls when they are styled and dry to seal in the benefits and moisture from the products you've already applied. Don't put oils or oily serums on your curls first, as this will not allow the other products to penetrate the hair and do their job. If, for example, you are using a gel, the oil will prevent the gel from penetrating the hair to encourage curls to form. If you'll be using a gel with drying ingredients such as alcohol, a leave-in conditioner (or a little conditioner left on your hair during your final rinse) will act as a base and provide a buffer against the drying effects of the alcohol.

A leave-in conditioner, specifically labeled as such, is a product to be left in the hair. It should be the first product you put on your curls after washing and conditioning, after removing a little moisture from your curls as explained in the Moisture Level Test section (p. 68). Don't get lazy and mix your leave-in conditioner with a gel, for example, in your hand. A true leave-in has ingredients and properties designed to benefit the hair when *left in* the hair. You must therefore layer your products properly: using a gel, for example, over the specially designed leave-in conditioner will actually seal in the beneficial ingredients of the conditioner. As the curls dry, they are protected from the heat of the sun or dryness in the air, etc., by the gel layer.

To get these products to work properly—whether you're a one-product curly or five—you must also learn how to section your hair. It's just one more step to get you to reach your true curly potential. Teaching you all these steps is like putting pieces of a puzzle together. Each piece (step) I share with you will make a beautiful curly image when put together. Miss a piece and your curls will be incomplete. Get these steps down and you'll never go back to lazy styling, knowing how great the curly style is when you put in the effort, especially when it gets you more styling days out of your curls.

Sectioning Your Curls

Let's face it, as a curly, we will always have a little frizz at times, but it's part of the curly personality! But hydrated, well-defined curls trump all in the curly world, so let's start with learning how to section hair to achieve the best results for our curly lifestyle hair goals.

Always start with hair that is clean (washed with sulfate-free shampoo or co-washed) and conditioned. Depending on the texture of your curls, you will have:

- rinsed off all your conditioner, for fine wavy hair or 2 curl pattern
- left in a little conditioner, for thick, coarse, wavy 2 curl pattern
- left in up to 25 percent of the conditioner, for 3 curl pattern
- left in up to 50 percent of the conditioner, for 4 curl pattern

Before you apply your styling product, it's important to detangle your curls. After you have cleansed your hair, finger rake to detangle your curls or use a wide-tooth comb before moving to a smaller tooth comb or brush, if you choose. When detangling, if you come across a knot or tangle, apply extra conditioner into the knot and massage in, then use your fingers or comb to work your way up from the bottom of the curly ends to the knot to detangle. If you have longer or thicker curls, you can divide your hair into large, pie-shaped vertical sections from the crown down to the neck to make detangling easier, using a clip to hold aside every completed section.

The average curly style will require three sections when applying styling product. A section will be 2-3 inches wide for medium-texture hair. For very thick or coarse hair, you may have 5-7 sections. Once you section your hair, you'll be working in subsections about the width of your hand, comb or brush.

You can try to save time by avoiding sectioning and applying your product everywhere, hoping you have evenly covered each curl, but you'll actually miss a lot of curls that way, get frizzy results as well as curls that don't have the same bounce as the curls with product on them. Choose a lazy way and you will get a lazy style. For best results, take the time to section the hair for not only a better curly style, but better next-day curls, too. If you put in the extra time on your wash and style day, you won't have to do it so often because the curly style will hold, saving you time in the long run, so it's definitely worth it!

You can also assess the whole curly picture before you section your hair. Your curls may be hydrated everywhere but the top layer, so you will know that when you get to the top section, you will have to mist with water from your spray bottle and maybe add a little leave-in conditioner to that top layer only, to help provide more moisture to that dry area. You may find the lower sections closer to the base of your neck to be smoother to the touch as you pinch down the strand, so no extra steps are needed there. But if you know you get really tangled at the base of your neck from wash to wash, then leave a little conditioner there.

If you're using only a gel as a styling product but your hair is still feeling frizzy and dry, you may have to start leaving in some conditioner when you wash your hair to provide a base to get the smoothness you need, or use a little leave-in/leave-on conditioner. You have to learn to read your curls to give them what they need. Don't keep using the same methods over and over if you are not getting the results you want. You have to analyze your hair and seek a remedy to get the results you want by using the correct products and applying methods. As you start applying styling product to your curls, it is better to go over any area not sealed properly and that feels frizzy than to have to style your hair all over again the next day because you didn't take the time on your wash and style day.

> ***Extremely Important Note:*** *As you get into learning the routines, you have to keep your eyes open and observe. If your hair looks frizzy when wet—and oh yes, it can, you've all seen it—it will be 10 times more frizzy when it is dry. So make sure to remedy this with the proper moisture level left on the hair before styling, and use the correct product application method to smooth the frizz. Frizz is the cuticle raised up, looking for moisture. So when we are styling our hair, we want to use methods to provide moisture to that cuticle and smooth it down to get a great curly style with as little frizz as possible. With optimal moisture level and proper product application, your styling product will effectively penetrate the cuticle and act as a glue to keep that cuticle down flat as the hair dries. Products applied the correct way will be the glue that holds this whole curly style together.*

Begin with the Moisture Level Test (p. 68) and repeat throughout the whole sectioning process to make sure the curls are wet enough to properly apply your styling product. Before sectioning your hair, do a quick cuticle check (as explained on p. 81)—it's your frizz-buster prevention check! As you move up each section, applying your styling product, keep this cuticle check in mind and maintain the proper moisture level. Add water with your spray bottle as needed and smooth out the frizzy cuticles by applying your styling products with your method of choice: fingers, comb or brush.

Sectioning

Section 1 is from the base of your hairline to just below either ear. Working horizontally across the section, clip the hair above out of the way. Use your fingers or a wide-tooth comb to detangle the section again (this is done for each section). You're looking to feel for a smooth surface. If you feel little raised cuticles as you pinch down the strand, keep running your fingers down, pinching the strand until you feel that smooth hair canvas. Apply your styling product with your fingers,

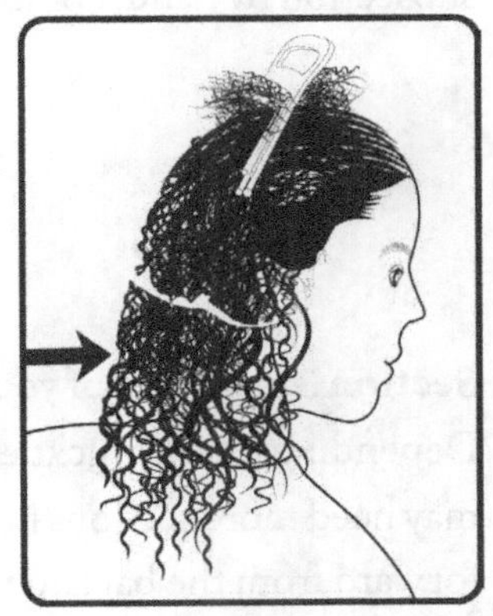

Section 1

starting from just below the root; avoid getting product on the scalp. Take sections no wider than your hand, and use your fingers, comb or brush as you work across each subsection. Make sure you do the same steps with each layer of product you use. For example, if you are using a leave-in conditioner, apply this first, using fingers, a comb or brush, then apply your second product, a gel, using the same method as for your first layer. Again, if you choose to use your fingers to apply styling product, continue running your fingers through your curls with the product in each subsection until you feel smoothness down each strand. As you apply your last layer of product, scrunch the hair as you go, lightly creating a fist of curls in each subsection, holding them from the ends up to the roots. Always make sure the curls have the proper moisture level before applying your styling product, and be sure you use enough product to coat each strand.

Note: I used a Pik to section the hair, but you could use clips.

Section 2 is from the lower ear to the partial ridge **(which you can see in the diagram)** just below the top section of your head. After detangling, rake your product through each subsection by hand, comb or brush, as above.

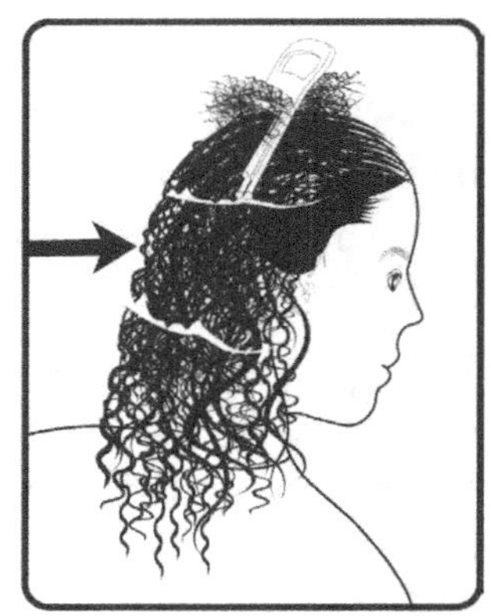

Section 2

Section 3 is the top of your head, the crown. Depending on the thickness of your hair, you may need more sections in the crown, moving forward from the back to front. Use one-inch subsections for very thick hair, two-inch sub-sections for medium to fine hair. Apply styling product to each section, moving forward from the back of the crown to the front hairline.

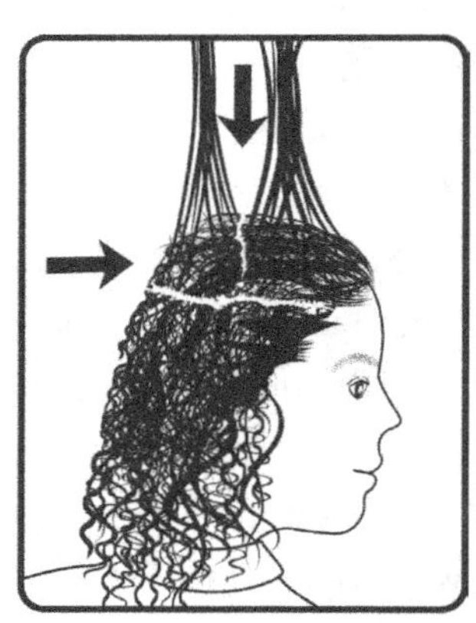

Section 3

Note: If hair is very thick at the crown, break Section 3 into 2 sections.

At the top sections, for those of you not averse to using a comb, first apply styling products by hand, then gently use an appropriate-sized toothed comb to distribute the product in all directions; comb it through the front, back, left side and right side. Twist the completed section of curls toward the back of your head and work on the next section, moving forward, sectioning the hair appropriately according to thickness until you reach the front hairline.

The next section goes into more detail on how to use your fingers, comb or brush to apply product so you can decide which method is best for you and your curly style.

Curly Tip

For a very frizzy and dry hairline, you may want to make sure you put some extra leave-in conditioner on your hairline. Place a small amount of leave-in conditioner on your hands and rub together; fan your hands as you smooth hair back away from your face. If you are fine to medium curly, simply take your styling product (if you're not using a leave-in conditioner) and use the same motion to effectively cover the hairline and smooth down the cuticle.

Choice of Method for Applying Your Styling Product

You can use one of three ways to apply product to your curls, or a combination of any of the three: by hands and fingers, by comb or by brush. This decision depends in part on what your personal preference is, but also, more importantly, on what your curls need. If you have really frizzy, dry hair, using your hands and fingers to run through your curls to apply your product will not get your styling product to penetrate the cuticles properly and will not result in the smooth surface you need to give you a better finished curly style.

Consider your outside layer of curls (I call the halo) on the top of your head. This layer protects your curls underneath, and is greatly affected by the sun and heat, cold of the winter, and other elements. It's every curly's wish that the halo would feel and look as nice as the lower layers. Well, this is why you may want to target this outside layer of curls with extra moisturizing and alternative application methods, such as the comb when styling your curls, to help with hydration. You can achieve almost the same results with your fingers, but it will take more time. The choice is yours.

Depending on your curly research, you may raise an eyebrow when I suggest a comb or brush for styling curls. I experience this reaction with many new curly clients. Most figure it's against curly rules to use a comb or brush. In almost every case, the curl clients I meet at the studio will shyly admit that they use a wide-tooth comb in the shower to detangle curls and help distribute conditioner, because they feel they can't work through their curls using their fingers. "Well, so do I," I tell them. "And I use combs and brushes on a lot of my clients as well." **So, why not use a comb for styling product, too, not just for conditioner in the shower?** Yes, I know, you may be thinking, "A comb for styling curly hair?" Using a comb is an effective frizz buster for my clients in the 2 to 3 curly patterns categories when applying products (conditioners included). My combo clients with 3 to 4 curly and kinky curl patterns are using paddle (or wet) brushes to effectively coat each strand when applying conditioner for the added benefit of deep penetration of both conditioner to the cuticle and styling product. Not only is combing a great frizz buster, it also makes applying your styling product quick! Better frizz control and a quicker styling routine. What curly would say no to that?

Again, let's clear up the misconception of using a comb or brush on curly hair. Using a comb or brush will *not*

1. make your curls stringy
2. ruin the curl pattern
3. break the curl

As long as your curls have the proper moisture level (which you have learned about in the Moisture Level Test section) when applying your products, you will find that your curls will retain the same curl pattern using a comb or brush as when finger raking your product through, but with better frizz control as a benefit.

When using your fingers to apply product to curls, you'll find in most cases the product won't penetrate the cuticles or provide the smoothness needed to make the raised cuticle lie flat, as a comb or brush can. The fingers can only smooth so many layers of the cuticle down the hair strand, but when you use a fine-tooth comb or brush, it's like 10 to 20 times more little fingers smoothing down your cuticle and effectively putting the styling product into each layer. You'll use less product, and it will also spread better using a comb or brush. That's not to say that if you prefer to just finger rake the product through, that you have to use the comb or brush method. You have to do what you feel is best for you and your curls. I'm here to open your curly mind to alternatives so that you can try another method if you're not getting the styling results for your curls that you're looking for.

Before you start applying your styling product, your curls must first be cleansed and/or conditioned and detangled. You can also do a quick "cuticle check," which is explained below.

Cuticle Check

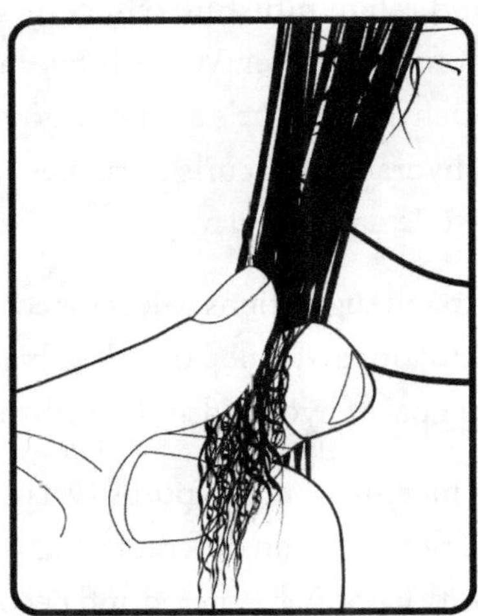

Pinch fingers down the strand to check for roughness / raised cuticles.

Do you want better-controlled curls with as little unflattering frizz as possible? What I want you to keep in mind as you are sectioning your curls and applying your styling product (as explained in the next chapter) is what I call the cuticle check. Right after you have cleansed and conditioned your curls, and before applying any styling product, see if you feel any roughness. To do this, you simply pinch a curl from root to end with your fingers and feel for any roughness down the strand. You need to create a smooth curly canvas before applying your styling product. Sometimes if curls are well into curl recovery, it's a matter of adding a little more conditioner and/or a little more water and running your fingers through your curls to smooth down the cuticle. If you feel a little roughness down the strand, you may want to implement the comb or brush method to help get the smoothness down the curly hair strand you need for a better finished curly style.

Porosity

Porosity is a characteristic of hair. Just as hair can be fine, medium or thick in density, it can also be described as *low, medium or high porosity*. Porosity determines hair's ability to absorb and hold water, which is worth paying attention to because moisture is so important to curls. Making hair healthy and able to absorb and retain moisture will contribute to healthy hair. Moisture in its purest form is water. Water is hydrating and is what hair needs to be healthy. Dehydrated curls are not a good look for anyone, so determining ways to hydrate your curls regardless of their porosity will result in a great curly style day after day.

Consider your porosity and suggestions below for conditioning, treatments and styling recommendations. It's all part of the big curly picture to help you work toward your goal of hydrated and healthy curls.

A curly can have low-, medium- or high-porosity hair. I've even met curlies with a combination of porosities on different areas of their head! A curly's low- to medium-porosity hair can be altered and become high porosity due to environmental factors (sun and heat), hot tools and chemical services (color and highlight services). Even treatments can affect porosity. Figure out which type you are, and choose the appropriate steps—which are outlined below—to work with that porosity.

If you have **low porosity**, you will notice your hair seems to repel water and it takes a really, really long time to get wet when you wash your hair. This is because the cuticle layer is closed so tightly and is so compact that it does not easily accept water. Products tend to build up as they just sit on top of the hair strands and do not penetrate the cuticle. Your hair can take a very long time to dry.

Using humectants such as glycerine, aloe or honey would do well on low-porosity hair because these products will draw moisture into the hair. Low-porosity hair does not react well with the use of protein treatments, as the proteins will simply layer on top of the hair strands and can make the hair feel drier and stiff from the buildup. These treatments can lead to breakage.

Low-porosity hair will more than likely require some work to get conditioners to penetrate the tightly packed cuticle layer of the hair. Low-porosity hair takes time to accept moisture, so work with smaller sections when going through your washing, conditioning and styling steps to help get better hydration and the best results. You will use products rich in emollients to soften the hair, and humectants to keep the moisture in.

The pinch and glide styling method (instructions for this method follow in this chapter) would work well for your routine for both conditioning and applying your styling product.

Medium-porosity hair is very easy to care for because the cuticles are lying closed, but not as tightly closed as low-porosity hair. Medium-porosity hair will easily hold water. If you have medium porosity, your hair will easily accept chemical processes such as colors and perms and highlights and will style easily. However, if over-processed and not taken care of, medium-porosity hair can become highly porous. Medium porosity can handle protein treatments occasionally, but daily use can weigh your curls down as they get over-saturated with excessive moisture. Medium-porosity hair can still be dry and frizzy to the look and touch, but adding a moisturizing leave-in is an easy way to fight dehydration.

Medium-porosity curls can choose any styling application method.

High-porosity hair can be a characteristic of the hair you were born with or can be the result of not being curl friendly with your routines. Your hair can look very dry and frizzy. It absorbs water quickly but cannot retain it.

Your hair tends to dry very quickly as well. Using poor-quality hair products or excessive heat styling and chemical services can severely damage the cuticle layer and affect porosity. Even environmental stress such as heat or sun damage can alter porosity. Each of these stresses alone or combined leave the cuticle layer wide open, exposing the cortex. Eventually, the cuticle gets eaten away and holes are left in the cuticle(s). The cortex is the soft center of the hair shaft and the cuticle is the hard, protective layer. The more damaging processes the hair is exposed to, the more holes there will be to the cuticle layer. This results in very frizzy hair that tangles easily due to all the chips and holes in the outer cuticle layer. When you compromise the protective outer layer—the cuticle layer—it's easy to understand why breakage to the hair strand occurs. There's nothing protecting the soft center. Even something as simple as going for a swim or washing your hair becomes a massive chore as hair tangles immediately upon immersion in water. So, if this is what you experience, doing a pre-shampoo (which is applying conditioner to your hair when dry) may help minimize the tangles when the water hits your hair on wash days.

Protein treatments will help seal and fill the holes in the cuticles, but they're not to be overdone, as too much protein can harden the curls and make them dry, brittle and frizzy. Do this once every week or two, depending on the curls' needs. Deep conditioning is different from a protein treatment, as deep conditioning provides moisture to the hair, whereas proteins repair. You should always seal a protein treatment with a conditioner to lock in the benefits of the protein treatment. Using anti-humectants to block excessive moisture from penetrating the cuticle to control frizz is suggested. Products containing ingredients such as beeswax, shea butter, hydrogenated castor oil, olive oil and coconut oil will fill and seal those little holes. Do not use these oils straight from a bottle from the grocery store. They aren't chemically formulated to be a hair product. You will learn more on oils in "Product Knowledge" and throughout The ABCs. Overall, high-porosity hair will be best served using leave-in conditioners and moisturizing styling creams to fill those holes in the cuticle layer. High-porosity hair craves excessive moisture, and these products, when layered, will provide this. If hair is high porosity as a result of poor curl routines, it will take some time and effort to repair.

The pinch and glide styling method would work well for both a conditioning routine and for applying your styling product. High-porosity curls can use any styling application method, but be very careful using comb and brush methods because of the fragility of your cuticle layers. Your hair may not be strong enough for this method, and you could experience breakage.

3 Ways to Check the Porosity of Your Curls

1. If you take a few strands of hair and put them into a bowl of water and the strands float, you have low-porosity hair. If your hair sinks immediately, your hair has high porosity. If you have medium porosity, your hair will slowly sink.

2. Alternatively you can pinch a few curly strands of hair from ends to roots (up the hair strand), and if you feel smoothness that means you have low-porosity hair. If you feel roughness that means your cuticles are raised and you have high porosity.

3. You can also take a spray bottle with water and spray on your hair. If the water beads on the surface, you have low-porosity hair. If the water sits on the surface for a moment or two before absorbing, you have medium porosity. If your hair quickly absorbs the water, it's a sign of high porosity.

   Note: Special consideration in part or whole can help with your curly routine if you know your porosity as we move through the "Styling Chapter." You can determine what styling application method is best for you. Remember that high-porosity hair has raised cuticles, and restoring the moisture back to your curls with the proper routines and methods will hydrate your hair and give you control over your curls. Low-porosity hair requires more effort to encourage water to penetrate the curls. Cleansing, conditioning and applying products properly to soften the cuticle for maximum moisture absorption is key. This will make sure products penetrate the hair shaft and don't sit on top of the hair strand, weighing it down and making hair dry, frizzy and brittle. Medium-porosity curls are the easiest to care for and style. Resolving frizz and dryness for this porosity type is very easy with adjusting routines. All the info you need to get you on your way is set out in The ABCs.

Compare Which Method Is Better for Your Curls

To compare the different styling product application methods, take two separate small sections of curls about an inch wide from the top (crown of your head). Apply your styling product (a leave-in conditioner is considered a styling product) on one section by finger raking through from close to the roots to the ends of the curls. Next, test the other section by first finger raking styling product through from close to the roots to the ends of the curls, then using a medium-tooth comb or brush on your curls. Pinch your fingers down each test section. If both sections feel smooth, then both methods will work. If you feel roughness as you pinch your fingers down the strands, your choices are to continue using your fingers to smooth and force the product in until you get the smoothness you desire, or use the comb or brush to get that desired smoother finish.

Choose one of these methods to apply your styling product.

Finger Application for Styling

If you want to strictly use your fingers and hands to style your curls:

1. Make sure hair is well detangled before applying styling product by raking through your curls from roots to ends with your fingers.
2. Keep hair wet and at the perfect moisture level, as previously discussed in Moisture Level Test section p. 68.
3. Section your hair according to its thickness (see "Sectioning Your Curls" diagram, pp. 77 & 78).
4. Use the correct amount of product in order of use (e.g., leave-in conditioner first).

5. Apply styling product to your palm and rub your hands together so your fingers are coated with the styling product.
6. Apply the product evenly down the curly hair section (as close to the root as possible, but avoid applying to the scalp) with your fingers.
7. Keep running your fingers through the curly hair section until you feel the curl is smooth.
8. You may have to work on one section, running your fingers through the hair a few times. Keep doing this until you feel your curls are smooth and effectively coated with the styling product.
9. If you are applying more than one styling product, simply apply on top of the first layer using the same method for your second layer of product. The second layer of product will go on quickly, because you have already provided a smooth curly section from the first product you applied.
10. Once you've finished applying product to that first section, gather up your hair (about the width of your hand) in that completed section from the ends and bring the handful of curls to the root; then scrunch to encourage the curl, if you want more curl. If your handful of curls is not making the squish sound I spoke of earlier, spray a little water and scrunch that section again.
11. Move on to the next section.
12. After you've applied all your products layer by layer to your whole head of curls, simply flip your head upside down and use a small microfiber towel to scrunch hair to the roots by the handful to encourage the curl.
13. Skip step 12 if you prefer a looser curly style. Leave the curls as they are without scrunching upside down with your hands or towel. The weight of the extra water not removed will help keep the curls down as they dry.

Comb Application for Styling

You'll have to decide which width of teeth for the styling comb will be best to achieve the smoothness you need. I like styling combs that are not too fine or too widely spaced: either a comb labeled "styling comb" or "men's grooming comb," and handmade, if possible. See comb styles in the "To Comb or Not to Comb" chapter.

First detangle your curls with a wide-tooth comb or your fingers, sectioning your curls as described above (pp. 77 & 78); apply styling product as shown below.

1. When using a comb to apply styling product, you must check the hair's moisture level as per the Moisture Level Test (p. 68).
2. Take the appropriate amount of styling product and apply to the palms of your hands; rub your hands together so your fingers have the product on them as well.
3. Run your hands evenly through a section of curls about the width of your hand with your fingers (get as close to the root as possible without applying styling product to the scalp).
4. Next, run the comb through from root to end at least two times down this section until you feel uniform smoothness down the curl. Make sure you comb both on top of each curly section and from underneath. This ensures even product distribution and cuticle smoothing.
5. If you find curls are knotted after raking the product through by hand, use the comb from the ends of the curl working back up to the knot and the root. (You will get rid of the knot more effectively this way.)

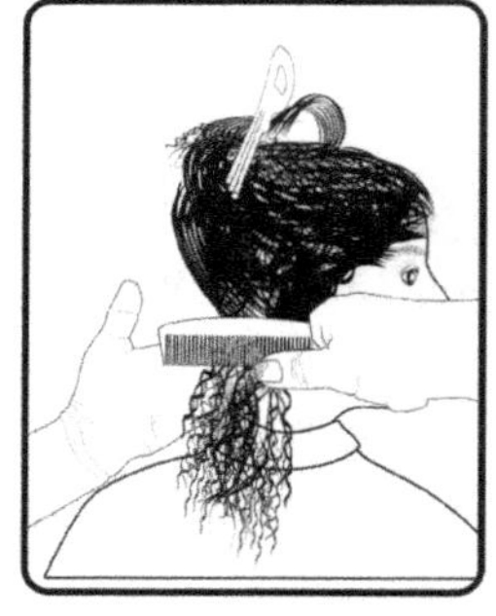

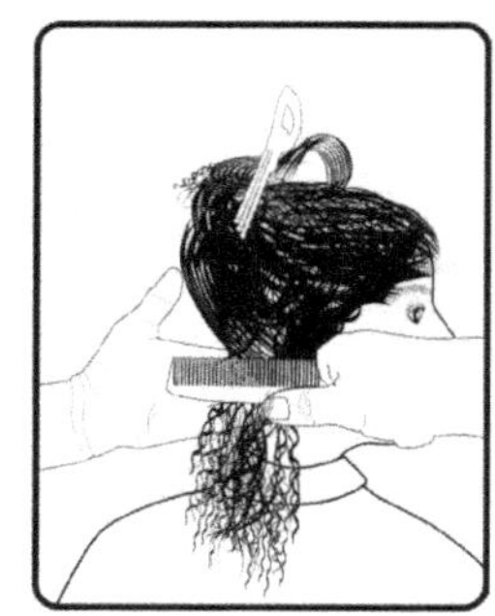

6. If applying another product in that section, use the same method as above, using fingers to apply and then combing through.

7. When the section is combed and coated properly, gather a hand-width of hair and scrunch curls from ends to roots to bring back the curl. If curls are not making the squish sound, spray a little water and scrunch that section again by the handful.

8. If the moisture check is done throughout applying your styling product, the curls will bounce back properly after combing the product in.

9. When you have applied all your products layer by layer to your whole head of curls, simply flip your head upside down, rake your fingers through your curls to re-clump them from the combing.

10. While your head is still upside down, use a small microfiber towel to scrunch curls by the handful to the roots to encourage the curl.

11. Skip step 10 for a looser curl. Leave the curls as they are without scrunching upside down with your hands or towel. The weight of the extra water not removed will help keep the curls down as they dry.

Brush Application for Styling

You'll have to decide which brush will work best for your curls. I opt for a paddle brush with soft bristles. Some curly clients like rubber bristles, like those found on a Denman brush.

1. Each curly section should be detangled by a wide-tooth comb or finger raking before you begin.

2. When styling with the brush, make sure the hair's moisture level is where it should be (perform the Moisture Level Test p. 68) so that curls can stretch properly when brushed.

3. Apply styling product to the palm of your hand and rub hands together to ensure your palms and fingers are evenly covered in product. A leave-in conditioner is considered a styling product and should be applied as your base layer, if using, especially for those with drier curls.

4. Run your fingers and hands down the curly section (a hand-width wide) evenly from close to the roots down to the ends with the styling product.

5. Use the brush to spread the product through for loose to medium curl patterns, brushing from midway down the hair shaft to the ends; then start back at the root and go all the way to the ends. This ensures a smooth, uniform surface and assists in detangling any tangled hair you may have missed initially with the wide-tooth comb. (For kinkier 4 curl patterns, I use the brush from ends to the roots, moving closer to the root a few inches at a time, then brushing through from root to end.)

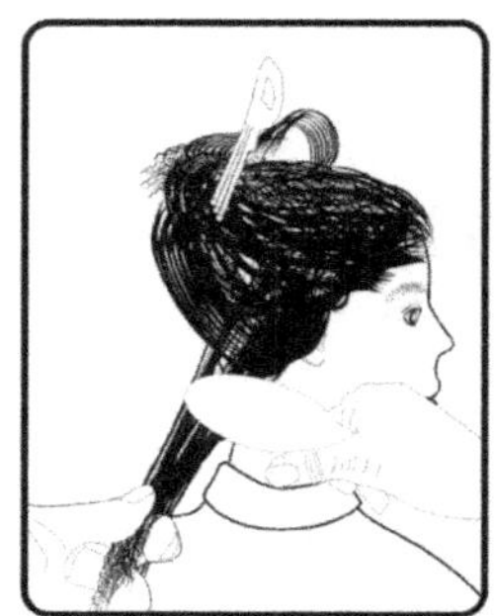
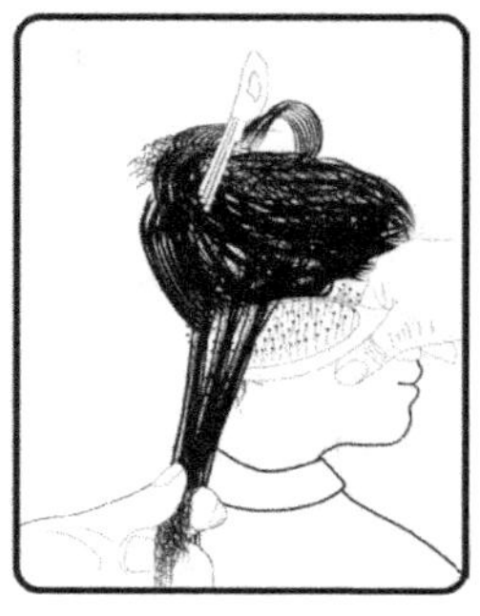

6. Continue to brush down the same subsection from on top and underneath that subsection until the curls feel smooth. This means when you pinch your fingers down a curl or clump of curls, you will not feel any roughness or raised cuticles (Cuticle Check, p. 81).

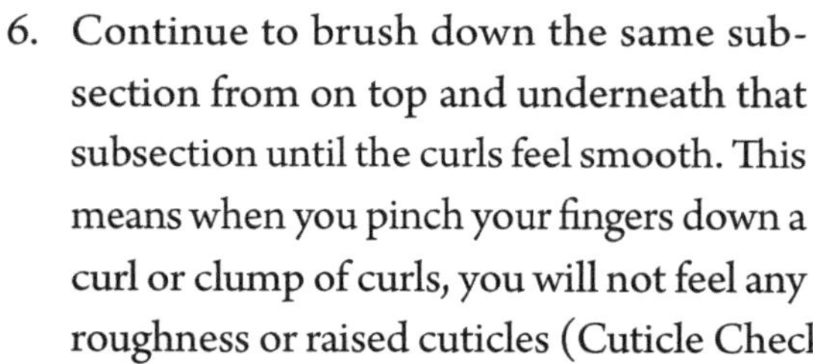

7. If you feel you need more product, or water to help spread the product, spray more water or apply more styling product by hand and brush through until smooth.

8. For very dry hair with really raised cuticles and a rough surface, you may have to run the brush through the section many times and then even continue finger raking to smooth down the cuticle.

9. If adding another product, apply it right on top of the completed section and brush through as above.

10. After completing the section, scrunch curls in small handfuls, gathering curls from ends to roots to reactivate the curl, making sure the moisture level is still optimal.

11. Continue with each section until your whole head of curls is complete.

12. Flip your head upside down, making sure the moisture level is still perfect; spray on more water as needed.

13. While your head is still upside down, rake your fingers through your hair to re-clump the curls from the separation caused by brushing.

14. Once you've encouraged the curls by scrunching and they are back to their normal state, hold curls by the handful to the root and squeeze well with your microfiber towel for the best curl encouragement.

15. Skip step 14 if you prefer an elongated curl. Keep head in upright position and simply rake fingers through curls, and don't remove any moisture with the microfiber towel. Leaving excess water in the hair, along with styling product, will provide weight to keep curls elongated.

Pinch & Glide Frizz Buster Method

Are you using your fingers to style your curls and not getting frizz-free results? When you do the cuticle check, can you feel the cuticles raised instead of lying down smoothly as they should? This styling method can be used to create smoothness in any area that needs a little extra care and hydration, such as that notoriously dry crown area or anywhere you need frizz control. You may like the results so much you end up using this method for your whole curly styling routine from nape to crown!

1. Apply your styling product.

2. Take half a thumb-width section of curls or a curl grouping (one clump of curls) from the frizzy area you are trying to hydrate.

3. Use your index finger and thumb to pinch down that section to create a smooth curly strand.

4. You may have to pinch and glide down the strand more than once to achieve smoothness.

5. Remember, you're looking to feel and see a smooth frizz-free finish. You shouldn't be feeling any roughness from raised cuticles.

   Note: *If hair is frizzy-looking when it is wet, it will be 10 times worse when dry, so take your time!*

6. Again, always keep hair wet and at the perfect moisture level, as previously mentioned in the Moisture Level Test (p. 68).

7. Don't worry. You're not straightening your curls. You're super-hydrating and making them smooth.

8. See step 12 of the Finger Application Method (p. 86) or Scrunching and Setting the Curls (p. 94) to reactivate your curls.

9. If your curl pattern is a 3 or a 4 and prone to frizz, simply let the curls rest and skip step 8 above, as your curls will more than likely have bounced back.

10. If you are a wavy (in the 2 range), just scrunch with a wet microfiber towel to encourage your curls.

> *Note: The pinch and glide frizz buster method is basically using the cuticle check (p. 81) as the motion to apply your styling product and achieve a balanced style with all your curls uniformly hydrated from the top of your head to the nape.*

This is a great method to provide ultra-hydration for curls with low porosity. Exceptional results can also be gained for high-porosity curls that need extra frizz control!

Curly Tip for Super-Thick, Extra-Dry or Kinky-Curly Patterns

Section your hair and completely detangle before applying your styling product. Always make sure your curls' moisture level is correct—even a little more wet than what I have suggested for other curl patterns. For those with 3 to 4 curl patterns (curly or kinky hair), if your hair is not wet enough when you apply your styling product, you may see a milky residue on the surface, because your styling product has not been absorbed properly. Keep a spray bottle handy with water, or with a tablespoon or two of conditioner and six ounces of water to mist on your hair when applying your styling product, and keep hair at the proper moisture level before applying any styling product, including leave-in conditioners.

For all the methods above, if you find your hands are sticking too much to your curls when you are scrunching for curl encouragement, simply do this step with the wet part of the microfiber towel only. I say "wet part," as I assume you have taken at least one squeeze of moisture out before you begin styling. The wet part of the towel will remove less product and provide more frizz control when scrunching.

For curlies in the 3c to 4a, b and c categories, I generally do not remove any moisture at all with the microfiber towel, instead allowing the curls to absorb all the moisture, because these curl patterns require the most moisture.

The next section will review how to finish your style, focusing on the scrunching steps mentioned above, and explain how to create your part. *Scrunch and set when hair is super-wet! A beautiful curly style is what you'll get!*

ABCs Flashback

Remember the elasticity test you did at the beginning of this book? If you noted which sections were drier, where the curl may be looser, this is the time to focus on using the correct products in those sections where you are trying to restore health. If your sides, for example, are a looser curl pattern from being pulled back in a ponytail or you just so happen to have a looser pattern there naturally, use a foam, light mousse or spray gel on those areas and scrunch really well with the wet part of your microfiber towel to encourage the curl. Or, if the hair at your crown is very dry, then target that area with moisture by leaving more conditioner in that section, or apply a leave-in conditioner to balance out your style. Get to know your hair needs in different sections and apply what's needed to get the best style results.

> **Note:** *Refer to "Pinch & Glide Frizz Buster Method" to help you with your frizzy crown! It's a sure-fire method to make those cuticles lie down!*

Scrunching & Setting Your Curls

If you have used a comb or paddle brush to apply your product, you will not lose your curls or ruin your curl pattern. We use these methods to create a frizz-free curly style. To encourage the curl back from all the finger raking, combing or brushing, which will have loosened the curl pattern, simply put your head upside down and rake your fingers through your wet curls. The moisture level should be hydrated according to the moisture

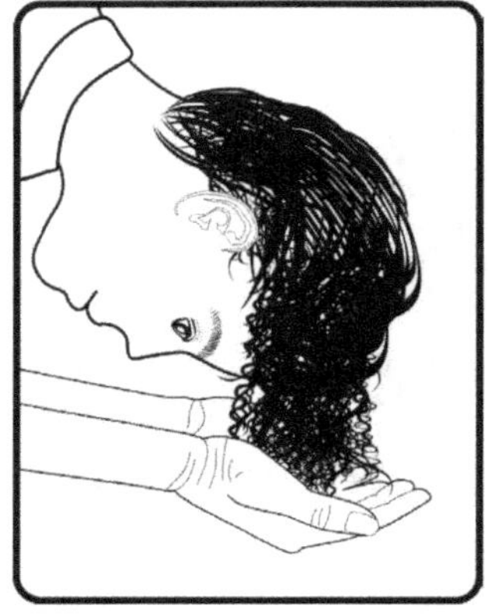

level test. If your curls' hydration level is not where it should be, add more water or conditioner and water from a spray bottle.

- With your head flipped upside down, use a catlike pawing motion with fingers spread apart, raking through all your curls two to four times. This will re-clump your curls; the wider the fingers are spaced, the wider the clump will be. Begin scrunching the hair by the handful with a closed fist to the roots and hold for a few seconds. This process will encourage and lock in the curly set. To recap this step, you are basically collecting a section as wide as your fist when closed and drawing the hair to the scalp, holding it, then releasing it and moving to the next section.
- Tip your head sideways and use the same process on each side.
- Scrunch more in areas where you find your curls may be looser.
- Slow and gentle is the name of this game.
- If you want a more put-together or clumped curl, scrunch your curls with gel in your hands.
- Next, take the wet part of your microfiber towel (the portion of the towel you will have used earlier to remove moisture before applying your product) and do your final curl encouragement, scrunching curls up to the roots by handfuls with the towel.
- These methods will leave hair more wet than you are probably used to, so you will have to see what drying method you prefer and

choose your washing days and times to allow for your proper curly drying time.

- Now that you've scrunched your curls, it's time to set them. Once set, you can let your hair air-dry or opt for one of the other drying methods described below.
- Next, gently flip (a big flip will stretch out your curls) or roll your head back from upside down to an upright position and shake your head side to side to allow a natural fall. The less touching with your hands you do from this point until your hair is dry, the better. You don't want to rough up the cuticles and cause frizz.
- For finer hair or curls that are resting closely on the scalp, simply use a tail comb to gently pull curls out and let them hang loosely.
- Gently lift the hair with the tail comb to define your part or let your curls fall where they may after gently flipping to the upright position and use your natural part. Another option is to keep head tipped back, allowing curls to fall back and have no part.
- If you have very short pieces at the nape of your neck because of breakage or regrowth, simply rake your fingers gently at the base and pull the curls down to elongate.

If you wish to add volume, please read the next section. Otherwise, skip to "Drying Your Curls" (p. 101). Once hair is dry using your method of choice, place a little pomade or a few drops of oil on your palms (so your dry hand doesn't stick to your hair and cause frizz); gently gather your curls into a ponytail at the top of your head (no matter how short your hair) and give curls a good squeeze all the way down the hair from root to end of that ponytail to get rid of the coating and hardness from the product you have used. Some styling products leave a cast on the hair as it dries and this motion will break the cast formation.

If you like the look of looser, fuller curls instead of a clumped-together curly look, shuffle hair at the roots. Spread your fingers wide, resting on the scalp to open the curl for fullness. Or simply squeeze hair section by section, gathering curls by fistfuls to loosen. Otherwise, let your curls be for a more put-together finished style.

Curly Tip

I quite often let my freshly washed, dried and styled hair rest for the day and don't squeeze, scrunch or shuffle my hair for quite a few hours, even after my hair feels like it is totally dry. I find I get better second- and third-day hair this way. A lot of curly girls with kinky curls also do this for better day-after-day curl.

Adding Volume with Clips

There are a number of ways to add volume when styling your hair. All curlies hate when the part line or the top of the head lies flat. Wavy girls feel their hair always looks triangular if their hair sits at the shoulders. There are a number of methods you can try to add lift and volume at the roots as your hair dries.

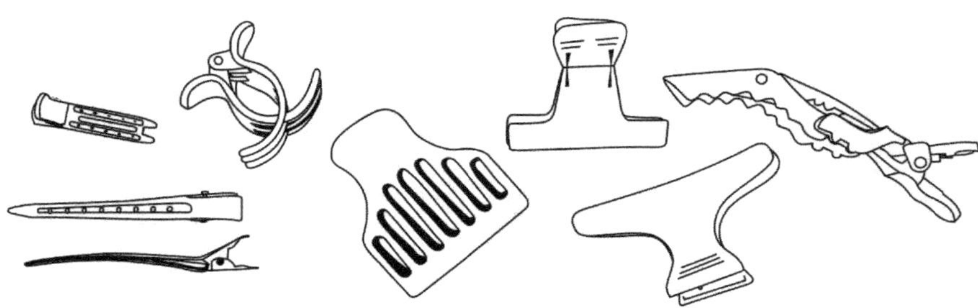

Clipping Method

You can use either single- or double-prong metal clips to achieve lift at the root. The single version (called a duckbill clip) will not give as much lift as the double-prong clip, but you will use fewer clips using this duckbill clip. The duckbill clip is also better for finer hair textures that can't hold the weight up of the double-prong clip, which is shorter and wider.

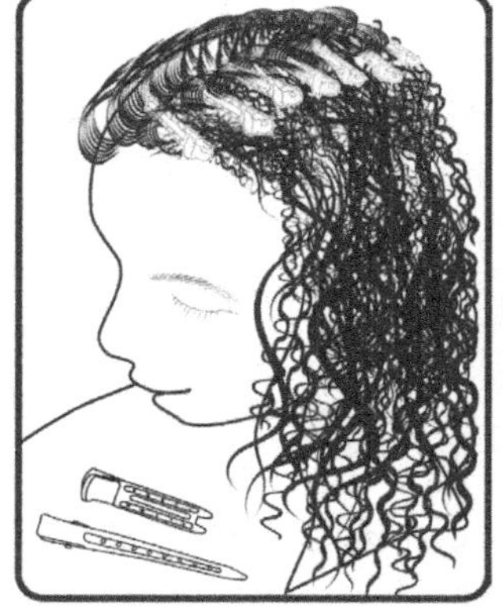

Preparing to Clip

After applying your styling product, and flipping your head upside down to scrunch your curls with a microfiber towel, make sure you take extra care to hold the hair at the roots at the top part of your head (crown) where you want to add volume while still in the upside down position. This will encourage a good lift and will make it easier to put the clips in.

The **single-prong** (aka duckbill) clips have a slight curve in them. When you use these clips, you want to make sure the curve faces to the back of your head so the curls flow back. The goal is to move from the back of the top of your head where your curls fall back over the farthest part of your head toward the front hairline. Even if your part line is not straight but rather random, or is diagonal or zigzagged, you're going to be putting the clips in the hair across the part line. This means a portion of the clip is going to rest across both sides of the part.

- Take the clip and rest it with the curve facing toward the back of your head, with one side of the clip resting on the scalp just off to the side of the part line.
- Open the clip (approximately one-third of an inch) and slide in the clip so it crosses the part line (opening the clip too wide will cause the clip to lie flat on the scalp instead of its edge: you want the clip sitting perpendicular to the scalp). If your hair is very fine, you may wish to connect two clips together (putting the clips in from both sides), which will lock them together and help keep them supported in the upright position.
- Keep inserting clips across the part line about one inch ahead of the previous clip, stopping about a third of an inch from the front hairline; otherwise, when hair is dry, you might see where the clip possibly left a dent in the hair.

Curly Tips

When inserting the clips, you may have to use your free hand to lift the curls on the opposite side to where you are inserting the clip to have balanced lift on both sides of the part line. Keep the clip closed and pointed at the root where you want to insert the clip. Then open the clip to slide in across the part line. Ensure you are not opening the clip too wide. This will help you clip the proper amount of hair in each clipping section. Opening the clip too wide off the scalp will grab too much hair and you will find it difficult to remove the clips when hair is dry. To provide maximum root lift, insert clips under the curls where they are visibly gathered or clumped together in a group. Refer to online resources and you will find many videos about how to do this method various ways.

Make sure you prepare to clip your hair as outlined above. For the smaller **double-prong clip**, still start at the back of your head, the crown; holding a little curl clump near the part line, affix the clip's open end on an angle downward toward the scalp. You might use anywhere from 8 to 14 clips to get the lift you want in the places where your hair lies flat on the crown, or any areas around the part line. Work your way toward the front hairline and stop about one inch from the front hairline; otherwise, you might see where the clip possibly left a dent in the hair.

You can use the clipping method anywhere you want to add volume or correct areas at the back of your head where you may have a split crown. Simply apply the clips to those areas and direct the curl (hair) over the clip. You can also add volume without having a part line at all. It all depends how you direct your hair back when applying your styling product. I like to use a horseshoe pattern on the crown to give a nice uniform roundness to the shape. This will resemble a halo made of clips surrounding the crown.

Adding Volume with Elongated Claw Clips Available in Various Styles

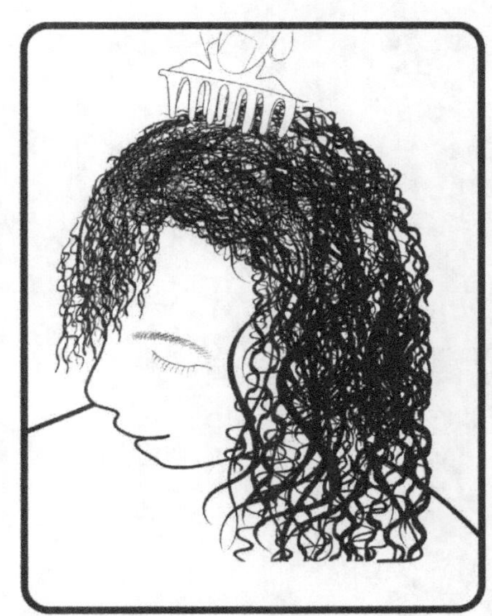

You can use these clips across the top of your head to add volume. Just choose the direction according to your part line and use as many clips as needed to provide lift. Usually four or five will do. Then either air-dry or diffuse until dry.

You can also use the clipping method to secure your bangs back from your face when drying your curls. Apply the clips with the open end at the hairline and gently insert clip through the curl so it rests on the scalp. You can rest the curl over the part that opens to support the hair when drying.

If you prefer to air-dry your hair, usually the clips will take about 10 to 20 minutes to set the style. Even if the hair is still wet when you remove the clips, the lift should be enough to add volume at the roots. If you're not happy with the lift, you can re-mist the hair at the top with a little water and put the clips in again to set the style. There are a few more ways to add volume using a diffuser, hair Pik and even your hands, all of which are explained in "Drying Your Curls," next.

Chapter 8

Drying Your Curls

How you dry your curls can make a huge difference between a great look and a catastrophic failure, not to mention the waste of time and effort washing, conditioning and applying products properly. Your drying routine is your closer, your home run for a winning style! Each step you have learned along the way is very important on its own, but this is the glue that holds it all together.

So, how should you dry your curls? So many options: natural air-dry, hair dryers, hooded dryers, diffusers or dryer mitts.

I've been asked many times what is the best method for drying hair. Just as curlies are particular with shampoos, conditioners, styling products and so on, so are they particular about how to dry their curly style. According to popularity, letting hair dry naturally (air-drying) wins hands down, with diffusing second in line; "plopping" is now becoming quite popular, too. If you've tried any of the methods included below before reading *The ABCs* and hated the results, I encourage you to try again, following the directions I have suggested here. I think you may find a difference.

If it wasn't for the fact that winters are typically so cold where I live in Canada, I would opt for naturally air-drying my curls year-round. With this method I find my curls are smoother and more well defined, and I get better day-after curls. Air-drying, however, does have its disadvantages. I feel that I look like a drowned rat with my curls stuck to my head during the drying process. Come on, curly people, we all know curls can take a long time to fully dry with this method. But, once the curls are dry, a little scrunch here and there, and turning upside down for a little fluffing and shuffling with my hands at the roots, and it's a good curly hair day!

Your drying method of choice will depend greatly on your lifestyle, schedule and timing. If a client is a no-fuss, no-muss curly, I suggest a good-quality hair dryer with a diffuser with little prongs on it. Tourmaline and salon-quality dryers are optimal for the best curly style. The heat that radiates from these tools is a lot gentler on the curls.

For those clients who have time in the morning but would like to multitask, I suggest a hooded dryer, as this allows the hands to remain free during the drying time for emails and so forth. My travel and on-the-road curlies definitely have to pack a diffuser when on the go, given that gyms or hotels generally don't provide them.

For the driving-to-work curlies in the colder months, natural air-drying using the heat of your car works great—it's like being in a body-sized hooded dryer! Just remember, if you are using the clipping method as described in the Adding Volume with Clips section (p. 96), make sure you remove them—all of them—when you get to work! In the summer months, keep the windows closed, as naturally air-drying with the wind blowing your wet curls around will not be a good look. For all the curlies with shoulder-length hair or longer, plopping is a wonderful method to dry and style curls; as you will learn, it's a versatile 3-in-1 method.

Diffusing Correctly

I have walked into many salons over the years to see this method being done incorrectly. Don't feel silly if you don't know how to diffuse your curls properly. Most professionally trained stylists don't either! Seems easy enough, though, right? Just point the dryer with the diffuser attachment at the hair and off you go, drying the curls. Not so! When I show my new clients how to diffuse their curls, they all admit they have been diffusing the wrong way. Either they position the diffuser on the ends of their curls, aiming the airflow to dry up the hair strand or flip their head upside down and start diffusing in this position when hair is soaking wet—all in attempts to add volume to the hair. What you get is volumes of frizz.

During diffusing, keep in mind the thousands of cuticles running down each hair strand. Diffuse correctly to control them. Whether you choose to dry your curls naturally or with a diffuser, adding volume with either a Pik or your hands, these are the steps to do in order to seal the cuticle to reduce frizz.

Sealing the Cuticle

1. Apply your styling products of choice.
2. Apply your hair clips for volume.
3. Keep your head in the upright position.
4. Make sure the diffuser opening (where the air flows through to blow on the hair) is at the top of your head of curls pointing downward (so the air flows down over the hair). The diffuser should be hovering directly over the crown approximately 3-4 inches from your curls.
5. Use medium heat and the medium airflow setting on your dryer.
6. Slowly move the diffuser along the hair from the top of the crown down toward the ends in a smooth motion for the first 2-3 minutes to encourage the cuticles to lie flat.
7. Do this all the way around your head, always working from the top down and aiming the airflow down the curls. This is your frizz-buster step.

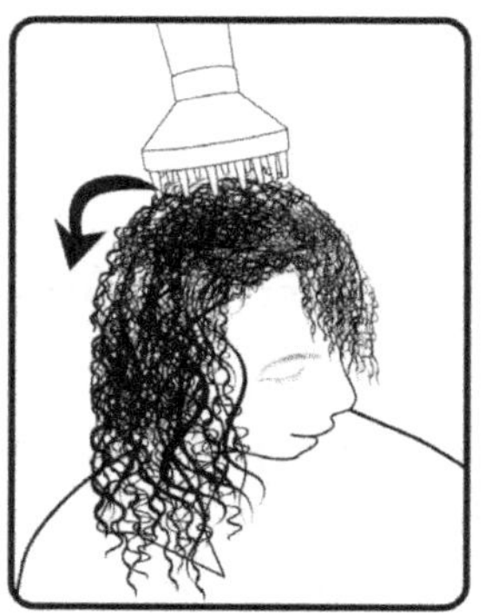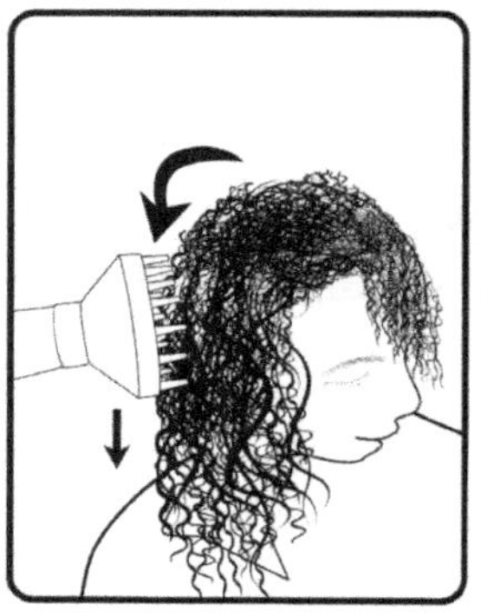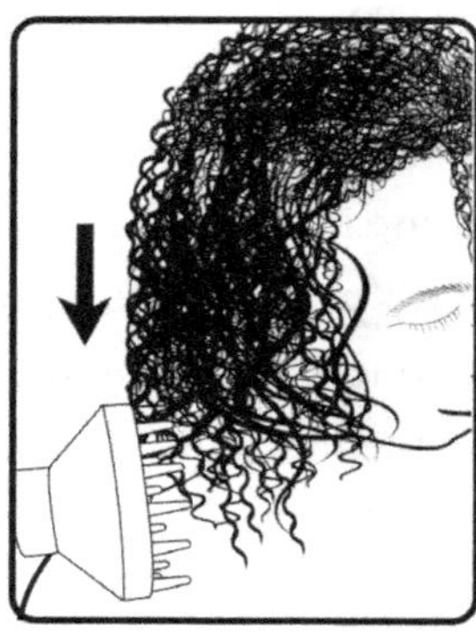

Move diffuser slowly down the curls from crown to the ends to seal the cuticles.

If you have used the right amount of styling product on your curls with the proper amount of water to provide moisture, the dryer will act as the catalyst to dry the styling product and gently seal the cuticle to the hair shaft. That's why I said earlier that this step is the glue that holds it all together. If you begin by immediately flipping upside down to dry your hair, and skipping this "sealing the cuticle" step, all the work you have done to get to the drying stage will be for naught. You will be drying the cuticle in a raised position, maximizing the frizz.

Natural Air-Dry

If you're a natural air-dry curly, stop at this step. Continue to naturally air-dry, as you've effectively sealed the cuticle and product has dried slightly to form a cast—you're good to go.

Hair Acrobatics

This is usually performed by long-haired curlies to add volume. There is a correct way to do this step:

1. Seal the cuticle as above for 2-3 minutes, depending on length and thickness of curls.
2. As soon as you feel the styling product begin to dry, flip your head upside down.

3. Cup sections of the hair in the teeth of the diffuser, using sections as wide as the diffuser head; gather from the ends and use the diffuser teeth to hold all the curls to the roots.
4. Hold that section to the roots for 15 seconds or so with hair dryer set at medium heat and medium airflow.
5. Press the cool-shot button for 5 seconds to seal the hair; if your dryer has no cool shot, just switch to the lowest setting for a few seconds.
6. Continue to dry that section over and over, 15 seconds using medium heat and 5 seconds with the cool shot until dry, then move to the next section to cup those curls, repeating the process. Focusing on drying one section at a time will reduce frizz and seal the curls better.

FYI, by cupping the curls into the teeth of the diffuser, you are taking the weight off the curls (the weight of the water, the styling product and even the curls themselves) while they dry, and are therefore encouraging the curl to dry in a tighter position for better curls. For wavy girls, this will work very well to maximize the curly wave.

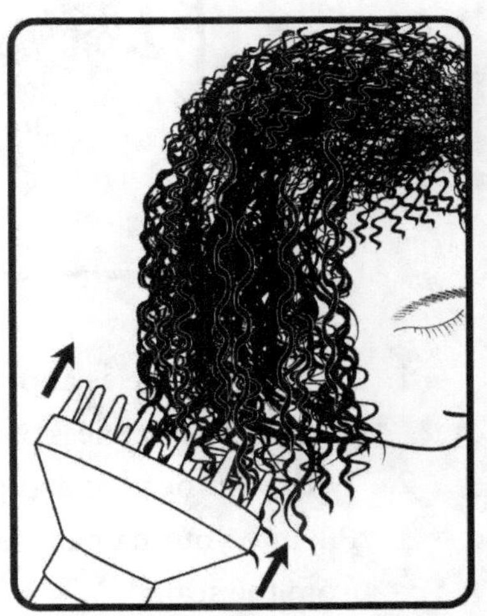

No-Volume Curly Styles

If you prefer as little volume as possible when diffusing, do not cup curls in the teeth of the diffuser. Simply press the diffuser lightly over the surface of the hair to dry, starting at the crown and moving down to the bottom of each section. Do not fluff or shuffle your hair at the roots when dry. To soften the product cast, gently squeeze the hair in small handfuls down each section from crown to end.

Adding Volume with a Pik

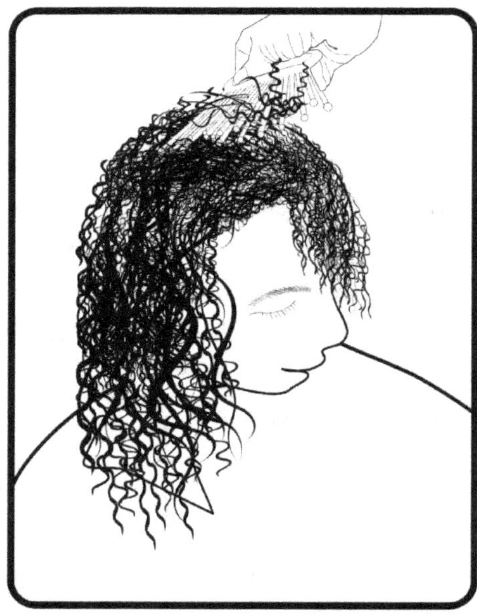

1. Seal the cuticle as above (p. 103) for 2-3 minutes, depending on length and thickness of curls.
2. With your head in an upright position, add volume by inserting a Pik into your hair at the roots, lifting curls one-half to two inches from the scalp.
3. Position the diffuser about 3-4 inches above your head, at the crown.
4. Use medium heat and the medium airflow setting to diffuse.
5. Hover the diffuser above where you have the Pik raising the curls and dry the hair.
6. Seal each section for 5 seconds with a cool shot in between.

Adding Volume with Your Hands or Microfiber Glove Designed for Hair

That's right! You heard me, use what you were born with!

1. Seal the cuticle as above for 2-3 minutes, depending on length and thickness of curls.
2. Apply a light layer of curl-friendly oil or serum to your hands so they won't stick to the hair and cuticles. Obviously no oil is needed on your hands if you are using a drying glove.
3. Use medium heat and the medium airflow setting to diffuse each section for 15 seconds, followed by a 5-second cool shot to seal the curl.
4. Whether you're upside down, tipping your head sideways or upright, gather a handful of curls, no wider than your hand can hold, and point the diffuser at your clawed hands so the heat can go through your hands.
5. Take your time doing each section to minimize the amount of time you're spending touching your curls. So, if you have to do the same section over two times with two cool shoots in between, you may find you get a better result.

For all the methods above, dry curly hair until it's **100 percent dry**. Some curl patterns don't like to be dried completely and get frizzy when they are, so watch for signs of frizz and stop diffusing at that point. If at the end of diffusing your hair you have any unsightly frizz or flyaways, just use a light mist of curl refresher to calm the hair down, or a very light mist of oil or shine spray.

Let curls rest anywhere from 15 minutes to a couple of hours, depending on the thickness of your hair. The thicker the curls' density, the longer I let them rest. Generally tighter and thicker curl patterns stay wet for hours or even for a day. For curlies who really want better next-day hair, save the steps on the next page until the next day if your hair takes longer to dry. Chances are you cleanse and co-wash your hair infrequently and get more styling out of your hair, so a curly hair rest and set day will work well for you.

Last Step: When Curls Are Completely Dry

1. Gently scrunch, or squeeze, your curls to the roots, cupping them in your hands to break the product cast. If you like more put-together curls, you can stop at this step.

2. Alternatively, to loosen up and open the curls and add volume, grab your hair in a ponytail at the top of your head, no matter how short and scrunch the hair all the way from the root down to the end of the ponytail to break the product cast. If you're a pomade or oil curly, put a light layer on the palms of your hands when you do this step.

3. If you want volume and separated (opened) curls, spread your fingers apart and place your fingertips at the roots and shuffle the hair to loosen the style and open up the curl, shuffling your hands all over your scalp in small sections the size of your hand either with your head upright or upside down.

   Note: *Use curl common sense. If, during the diffusing, curls start to go frizzy, simply stop and air-dry the rest of the way or use the plopping method.*

"Mermaids" are curlies with hair past their shoulders who want volume. Good coordination is required to do this, but more likely also someone like a sibling, friend or significant other to help!

1. After properly applying all your styling products, roll up a medium-sized towel that will be used to prop your head at the end of your bed.

2. Lie down, with the nape of your neck resting on the towel; your hair will be cascading like a waterfall down the edge of the bed.

3. Dry your curls in a downward motion along the hair shaft for 2-3 minutes to close the cuticle or until you feel your hair product begin to set (in most cases, you'll need someone to help you diffuse this way).

4. Then, cup hair section by section into the diffuser teeth and hold to the scalp for about 15 seconds.

5. Apply a cool shot or lower temperature for 5 seconds to cool curls down; release hair and move to the next section, or keep doing this sequence on the same section until dry to maximize curl and reduce frizz.

6. When hair is 100 percent dry, do steps 1 to 3 as above, **Last Step: When Curls Are Completely Dry,** according to your preferred method to break the product cast and loosen curls, add volume or keep curls intact.

   Note: *Never use what I call the "accordion motions"—opening and closing the gap between the length of your hair and roots over and over to dry. You are to simply hold the hair in one position and release. Doing a lot of unnecessary up and down motions while diffusing will just break the seal of the styling product you have used to reduce the frizz and instead create frizz; you will not end up with controlled, defined curls.*

That, my curly friend, is the way to dry your curls properly.

Plopping

Plopping is a versatile method, as it can be used for three separate styling routines.

- To protect your curly hairstyle when sleeping.
- As a curl refresher method. When curls are looking a little frizzy, lightly mist hair with a curl refresher of choice, and follow the steps below, plopping curls for 15 minutes to allow to dry.
- To style from a wet-to-dry method, as described below, with freshly washed and conditioned hair with styling product applied.

How to properly plop your hair:

1. Use a lightweight cotton or preferably thin jersey T-shirt to plop.
2. Flip your head and your curls upside down and allow curls to rest in the middle of the shirt.

3. Twist the sleeves so they wrap around your head and tuck them in (there are a number of methods online to choose from); curls are "plopped" and protected on top of your head in the little pocket you have created within the shirt while you sleep.

4. In the morning, remove the shirt and let your curls rest a bit so they can fall from the upright position of being plopped.

5. If the curls are still damp, diffuse with medium heat and medium airflow until hair is 100 percent dry.

6. Or if curls were plopped dry and you used this method to protect curls at night and you find your curls looking frizzy, lightly mist water, conditioner and water, or curl refresher on your hair.

7. After misting hair, simply graze the palms of your hands down the outer layer of your curls to calm any curly frizz that may have occurred overnight.

8. Read your paper, have a tea or do your makeup, and your curls will go back to where they were the day before in a few minutes.

9. Then follow steps 1 to 3 of **Last Step: When Curls Are Completely Dry (p. 108).**

10. Shuffle the curls at the roots to fluff and wake up the curls from their resting place, or use a little pomade to define the curls and you're good to go.

11. If you're a wavy curl, lightly mist alcohol-free hair spray or spray gel on the outer layer to control frizz.

Plopping requires planning your washing routine to allow a drying period anywhere from two hours to overnight, depending on the length and thickness of your curls. This method takes the weight off your curls while drying—gravity causes the curls to drop, as with air-drying—yet still allows the hair to dry naturally and slowly, sealing the curls. Plopping is a great wet-to-dry styling method for longer hair, especially if you have a thick texture and wavy curl pattern; your curls tend to be curlier when first dried, but as the day goes on, the weight of your hair causes the curls to drop. This method will help encourage your waves, taking the weight off them as they're drying and keeping that curl pattern in a better position throughout the day once fully dried. Use an oversized lightweight jersey T-shirt for best results, because a heavy cotton T-shirt will pull out too much moisture and cause your scalp to become too warm and sweaty; sweating causes frizz if there is no airflow.

Crochet Hair Bonnet

This hair accessory is great to use for the wavy curl or curliest with super-long hair. Loosely pile your curls into the bonnet. Make sure you purchase the appropriate size for your hair length and thickness to hold the curls from hanging too loosely. They come sized from small to extra large. When hair is piled into the bonnet, it takes the weight off your curls to retain the curl pattern and encourage the curl when wet-to-dry styling. Wet curls left to hang dry

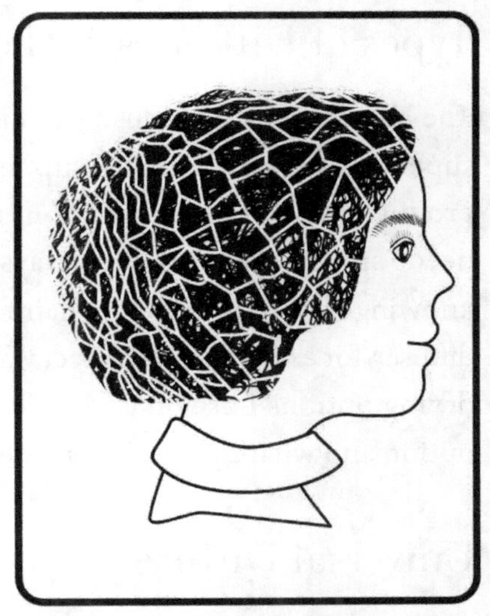

(especially thick wavy or extra-long curl patterns) will result in a looser wavy style. For an uplifting curly style use your root-lifting clipping method; then pile curls in the crochet bonnet and sit under a hooded dryer for maximum curl results, or allow to air-dry.

Curly Tips

- *When it comes to getting the best curly results, best to not touch curls when drying naturally. Less touching equals less frizz.*
- *If using a hooded dryer, a good trick to reduce excessive frizz on the top layer is to spray a small handkerchief with spray gel and place it on the crown, securing with a few pins or baby clips, to buffer the direct airflow on that area when drying while allowing the rest of the hair to dry freely.*

- *If you're experiencing frizz during high-humidity seasons when naturally air-drying your hair, try diffusing your outer layer for 2-3 minutes with medium heat and medium airflow (remember to direct the airflow down the hair strand). This will force down that little cuticle when the humidity is slowing the drying process; the cuticles will close down quickly and you can then let the hair dry the rest of the way naturally.*

Types of Diffusers & Hair-Drying Accessories

The hair and beauty industry is a multi-billion-dollar industry. With that super-huge playing field of suppliers comes the availability of so many products with numerous options for accessories to dry curls. Curly hair needs special care, but not always the most expensive gadget. It's about knowing how to prepare the hair for styling and how to use the gadget (a diffuser, for example) the correct way. Here you will learn about the different drying options I use on curly clients, what I feel is beneficial about each option and what to look for when choosing one.

Universal Diffusers

Natural air-drying seems to be the most popular method for drying curls, with diffusing close behind. Diffusers are first on the list here and can be sold alone or as an attachment with a hair dryer. Either can be effective—it's how you use it. Medium heat and medium airflow are the most important things to be mindful of. Anything too hot on curls is going to create frizz. If your hair dryer doesn't come with a diffuser and you decide to purchase a universal model, take your dryer to the store to make sure the diffuser fits, as universal diffusers don't always fit as advertised. If you find the fit of the diffuser isn't good and the diffuser pops off your dryer, use a heavy-duty elastic band, like those big fat ones used in grocery stores for banding broccoli together. Put this elastic on the end of the dryer and snap the diffuser on; you may need two overlapping each other to create a snug fit. I have never had an elastic melt, but it could get messy if your dryer does by chance melt the band. Check the heat resistance if concerned.

Also when choosing a diffuser, don't go short and compact when it comes to size. You want a diffuser with as long a shaft as possible. The farther the airflow has to travel to reach your curls, the less direct heat to push on the hair. This will dry the hair gently and seal your styling product properly, and therefore cause less frizz.

Hair Dryer with Diffuser Attachment

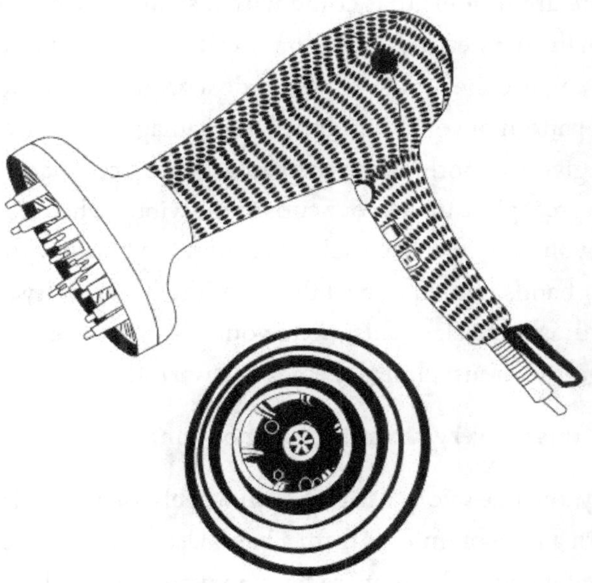

Folding Diffuser

Diffusers are available in different styles. Some come with teeth or little raised prongs on the end to hold the curls while diffusing; others simply have a vented end where you rest your curls to dry. Some diffusers even have a little cup at the end where the hair rests inside as heat is applied. I suggest purchasing the diffuser with the little teeth or prongs: they will assist in holding the curls when adding volume.

A good universal diffuser will cost around $20 to $25. There are inexpensive universal diffusers that fold (they're usually made of silicone and retail for $10 to $15), but their shafts are not long, and they do not buffer the airflow as well as the full-size, non-folding ones do. Use lower heat settings with the folding diffuser to dry your hair to make up for the shorter shaft.

Hooded Dryer / Hard-Top Dryer

I love this drying method for many reasons, but mainly because a hooded dryer gently seals curls as it dries when using medium-heat settings. Other benefits are:

- You can use this dryer for treatments that require heat.
- There are models that come with a steam setting. Some curlies actually like steam as a way to refresh second- and third-day hair.
- You can use the hooded dryer to do a great roller set to change the curl pattern of your hair in the least damaging way. Roller sets seal and give a smoothness to the hair that can't compare.
- It's a great place to dry your curls in the winter when it's cold outside and you don't feel like walking around the house with wet hair.
- Your hands remain free while under the hooded dryer, so you can multitask: check emails, write your to-do lists, read your favorite magazine or just chill and enjoy the warmth.

So all in all, this is a very versatile drying option.

You can buy one like salons use that is on wheels, or a model that sits on a counter with a base or unfolds from a base. Used retro ones can be found online and at garage sales that are fairly inexpensive. Pick one according to your space and budget. When using a hooded dryer, the setting should be at medium heat, or even lower if you are really prone to going frizzy during curl recovery. Curls may take longer to dry, but the hood tends to mimic the natural drying process. Because the air is gently going through the small holes—in most cases far away from the heat-producing source at the base—the curls are not being blown around with air force and this reduces the chance of excessive frizz. Another reason you should not use high heat is that the excessive heat will break the product seal on your hair cuticles and that will also create frizz. High heat and high airflow can also force too much air through the dryer, pushing your top layer down and making that section flat.

You can use the hooded dryer to get hair 80 to 90 percent dry, then let the hair air-dry the rest of the way as it cools down. Alternatively, dry your hair 100 percent and then set the dryer on the cool setting for 2-3 minutes to seal your curls. Test both ways to see which results in a better curly style. But always let the hair rest and get to room temperature for a few minutes, or use the cool setting at the end of the drying cycle. Only then, once the hair is dry, should you do your scrunching and fluffing if you choose, as you learned earlier in **Chapter 8, "Drying Your Curls: Last Step"—When Curls Are Completely Dry (p. 108).**

Price Points

I've seen second-hand hooded dryers for $20 to $25 at garage sales. New hooded dryers range from $75 for a tabletop model to $300 or more for one that you can wheel around.

Dryer Bonnets

These are now available in a variety of sizes. Some come as a single unit with heat settings and a hose connected to a bonnet; others are bonnets that connect by hose to your own blow-dryer. Bonnet dryers are great for curls needing treatments that require heat. The larger-sized bonnets will work well with roller sets. In some cases for different patterns (fine or medium-textured hair), the bonnet dryer may crush curls. Bonnets are an economical way to go if looking for portability and price.

Price Points

Dryer bonnets with a drying unit are upwards of $50, while I've seen dryer bonnet attachments as low as $10.

Dryer Sock Diffuser

To get similar results as a salon-quality blow-dryer, simply use a dryer sock on an inexpensive hair dryer. These accessories can't add volume the same way a diffuser with raised prongs can, but the airflow from the dryer is reduced, so it is perfect to gently dry your curls using radiant heat with minimal airflow. If you use the **hair Pik or hand method** (Chapter 8, "Drying Your Curls") to dry your hair or use clips to add volume, this drying method will work well, following the same diffusing method also found in Chapter 8 (p. 106), by going down the hair shaft with the dryer sock diffuser to seal the cuticle for 2-3 minutes. If you want a little volume, use your hands, coated with a light film of serum or oil, or cup curls in small sections in your hands to dry with volume and lift while aiming the dryer sock diffuser at each section. This accessory and method is good for all textures, but especially for finer ones, because it cuts down the direct airflow on the curls.

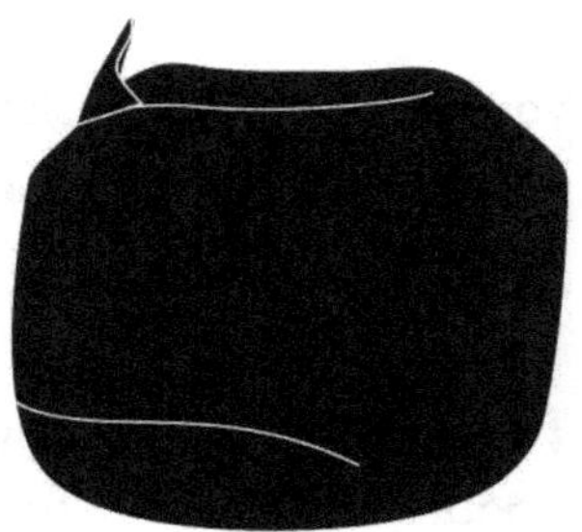

Dryer Sock Diffuser

Price Points

Dryer sock diffusers cost $7 to $15. So for a tight budget, this is the diffuser to get, especially for traveling or going to the gym. Another big plus for this low-priced accessory is that it fits most any dryer and is compact and light to pack.

Dryer Mitt

This is an accessory you put on your hand to help dry your curls. Usually made of plush microfiber, the mitt can be used to remove moisture from curls at the styling stage, or you can use it with your diffuser to dry the curls, with the mitt replacing your bare hands to minimize contact; some people feel that bare hands touching the hair creates frizz. My suggestion of lightly applying oil or serum on your hands first as previously instructed reduces this. The dryer mitt is a good option for those who don't want to touch their hair when it's wet. Wearing the dryer mitt, cup curls by the handful and apply heat from your diffuser.

Price Points

Dryer mitts cost $15 to $25, depending on whether it's a name brand.

> **Note:** *Never use a hair dryer on wet curls without a diffuser on it. The direct airflow on your hair is too harsh and will make your hair very frizzy. However, when hair is almost 100 percent dry, you can direct a dryer a few inches from the the root with the nozzle attachment to add fluffy volume to your finished curly style.*

Chapter 9

Sleeping Curly

We have a great style all day, but it's time to go to sleep. How do we protect our curly locks from pillow rub, knotting up and losing their shape overnight? The most important thing to keep in mind is that **our scalp and curls need to breathe when sleeping.** So many external and internal forces can affect us sleeping curly: the seasons, hormones and the temperature of our bodies constantly heating and cooling as we sleep. **We have to make sure when we protect our curls that we use a covering made of the right material, one that allows the airflow in and heat from our scalp to escape. If you are new to the curly methods and your hair is still going through curl recovery, you may not get the best next-day curls. Don't worry, your curls will show you the love by giving you better second-day hair as you change your routines and your hair gets healthier.** Use one of these methods below to help you sleep curly.

Plopping, as mentioned previously, is not only a great way to style and set the curls, but also a great way to protect your curls when you sleep. Mist water, conditioner and water, or a curl refresher on the curls that need waking up and follow the instructions set out in the Plopping section of "Drying Your Curls."

Loose braids work well for very thick or long curls. Do a large, loose braid before you go to sleep. It may change your curl pattern if you have finer hair, so don't make your braid too tight. I used to braid my hair while my hair was upside down so the braid end would rest at the top of my head. That way, the little curls at the nape of my neck were protected. Use two loose braids if hair is really thick; this also makes it more comfortable if you sleep on your side.

The **pineapple method** is a popular way a lot of curlies protect their curls when they sleep. This involves loosely piling your curls on the top of your head using a loose pony tie so you don't ruin the curl pattern. I prefer using a lightweight plastic claw clip, as they don't seem to change the curl pattern the way hair ties do when you let your hair out. If you have a lot of curls, you may need two claw clips. Use one to hold up the front and side curls and the other to keep the curls at the back up. In the morning, your curls may react the same way as plopped curls, with the curls sticking up from being clipped up all night. However, within a few minutes after using a light mist of water, water and conditioner, or a curl refresher spray, the curls will lie back down.

Scarves work well, too, if the scarf stays put on your head when you're sleeping. Use a silk scarf if you want to tuck your hair up for the night. Silk is more expensive, but it breathes well because it is a natural fiber and is lightweight, allowing the scalp and hair to breathe.

DO NOT USE satin bonnets or bandanas, which have been ever so popular for decades for many a curly to protect their curls at night. Avoid these polyester-based materials that are available everywhere! You are suffocating your scalp and creating a frizzy incubator for your hair while you sleep, because these materials don't breathe. The only thing that makes this fashion statement worse is if you smother your curls in coconut, castor or olive oil … well, any oil! The combo is a truly dehydrating experience for your curls. Not only can your scalp not breathe (because of your combo satin bandana and oil-basted curls), neither can your curly strands. You will encourage a lot of breakage and split ends, and will be lucky to see hair growth at all if you're in the 4s curl pattern category! Your scalp and curls need to breathe at night.

The only exception I would make for wearing a satin bandana or bonnet is while you are cooking. You won't suffocate the curls in that short period and the satin will effectively buffer the odors and grease from penetrating the hair. Using a covering for your hair made from a natural fabric that breathes would allow airflow and odors into your curls.

That said, if you still feel the satin will work for you and want to try it because you have finer hair and you don't sweat or get hot at night, you can do so to save money (as these products are cheap), but if you see a lot of frizz or dryness on your scalp, toss them to the curb!

A **mesh bandana** is also a good option to use to protect your curls when sleeping, as long as you can see through the material. Even though these types of products are made from polyesters (unnatural fibers, like those the bonnet or other bandanas are made of), the holes in the mesh provide ventilation. That means there is a place for the air to flow through, allowing your scalp to breathe. A mesh laundry bag cut into a triangle, or an old basketball or sport jersey can do the same job. Be creative and think outside the curl box and you will come up with the perfect way to protect your curls when you rest if you're a DIY kind of curly!

Hair tubes are new on the market. These are basically elongated neck warmers usually made of a thin microfiber material. Again an unnatural fiber, but it's lightweight and allows the scalp to breathe. You put the hair tube over your head and pull it down onto your neck, then slowly pull the tube up from the opening at the top of your neck, so one end stays around your ears and the opening at the top has your hair resting through. If you find the hair tube slips when you are sleeping, you can secure it with pins or clips at the base of your neck and temples. Depending on the length of the hair tube and how much hair you have tucked in, the end of the tube can flop over and remain open, or you can clip it shut or tuck the end in at the front by your forehead; essentially, you're mimicking the look of TV cartoon character Marge Simpson, with her blazing blue hair all up in the air.

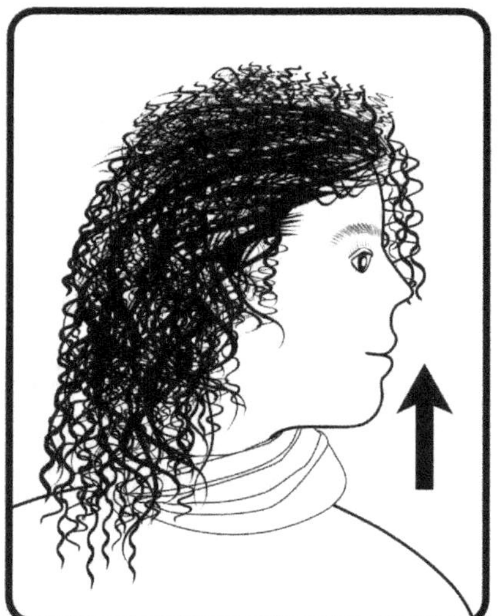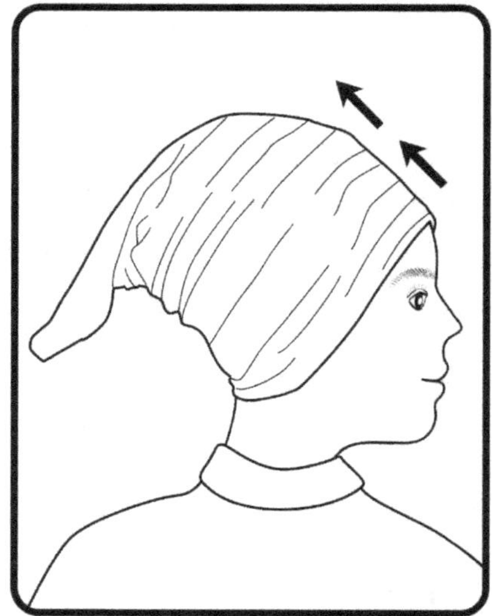

Put hair tube on like a neck warmer. Pull up over your head
and allow curls to rest loosely through the open end.

You can also make your own "DIY hair tube" from an old pair of microfiber tights or leggings. Use the ones made of the thinnest material possible. You don't want to have a thick, heavy hair tube, or again, your scalp will not be able to breathe properly. Simply cut from whatever width of the leg portion that will be suitable to accommodate the width of your hairline and make the tube portion as long as you wish up the leg as needed. Easy as that! While you're at it, use the full pair of tights and cut two hair tubes. Use the smaller portion of the legging down by the ankles to make scrunchies!

You can also use a pair of queen-size pantyhose to make a hair tube. Yes, this is quite possibly the oddest thing I have ever made to protect my curls. I left about 10 inches of pantyhose on each leg and cut off the rest. I pulled the waist support section over my ears and pulled the legs up at the top of my head and tied them once to secure. For my finer curls, the nylons didn't provide a good result, as the pantyhose really crushed my curls. A curly with thicker hair will be more successful with this method. Nylons are lightweight and easily accessible, and allow the scalp to breathe.

Pillowcase: A Resting Place for Your Curls

If you prefer to sleep with your hair free, any material that will help to reduce the friction of your curls against your pillow will help. When it comes to pillowcases, I know some curlies opt for one made of satin, because the curls just slip and slide easily on that material and won't tangle. Suffocating your curls when resting your head on the unnatural fiber isn't an issue at this point, because you're not wrapping your curls in it—you're merely looking for a smooth surface to rest your curls on.

A pillowcase with material that has a slight sheen will work, as it won't cause the friction that a standard type of cotton or, worse, flannel or fleece, pillowcase would; the likes of satin also won't draw moisture from the curls. If you want to invest a little more, a silk pillowcase is a perfect place to rest your head of curls. You can pay less and get a pillowcase made with a high thread count, such as percale or Egyptian cotton, which will work almost as well.

The Internet is a great resource where you will find many curly people willing to share step-by-step instructions on how they protect their curls at night. Take advantage of this resource to see how other curly people are doing varied methods of what I have set out above.

Chapter 10

The Kinky Curly Curl

I needed to devote a special section just to you, the most fragile of the curl patterns, who are always seeking moisture for their curls but are usually not finding a remedy, even after slathering your hair in oils and concoctions. This kinky curly pattern in the 4s category has the highest percentage of people using relaxers and chemical straighteners on their hair. Here's my chapter dedicated to help your curls be the best they can be!

I have seen many clients who have decided to go the healthy route for their curls, breaking the creamy crack addiction (relaxers/chemical straightening services). A lot of times, however, kinky curlies going clean end up exchanging one bad habit for another by turning into flat-iron junkies or adding braids and weaves to their routines. In the end, the hairline continues to recede and the curls suffer breakage and damage, because these routines are just as bad, and in some cases worse, as when using relaxers. The front hairline is the most fragile area on the head, so excessive heat from irons or tension from braids can compromise that hairline and create a recession that can't be turned around. Transitioning relaxed hair to natural is hard. The curl pattern will take time to show and grow in, and straight ends need to be cut off. The stages in between make it hard to style and look nice as the new curl pattern emerges. But there's no way around the transitioning: you have to go through the process. And I know it is a process.

Some curlies have been doing these routines for years and years, maybe their whole curly lives! Things have changed a lot in the curly world over the last decade or longer. With the advancement of hair care and knowledge of how to care for curls, going natural is simply a matter of finding what products and routines work well for your curls. Don't let your curls be trapped in the past curly bondage. This will not be an easy road; it will take time to get your curls to be where you want them to be. Years of damage from chemicals, straightening, blow-drying, pulling, braiding and trapping in oils with satin caps—your curls will need time to recover.

You must keep in mind, the tighter the curl is, the more fragile that hair is. All the bends and turns in the curl contribute to its fragility, so much so that some kinky curly hair feels like light fluff. It's a curl pattern so curly that you won't even see the pattern at all if you are using improper methods. The unrecognizable pattern can also have the appearance of steel wool. Your curls will look as though they never see growth.

If you're using shampoo, this dries out the curly hair so badly that your ends just break off. It's something you may not be able to see when it is happening, but they're breaking off between washes and blowing off into the wind. Or worse, once your curls are styled and dried, you can feel your curls breaking off between your fingers as you touch them. You may even think you have dandruff because of the flakes you see in your hair. It's really your dry ends that have broken off, settling on your hair, not dandruff. If you have concerns about it being dandruff, go to a doctor for your hair; the doctor will prescribe accordingly. DO NOT USE store brand dandruff shampoos: they are the worst possible product you could use for your curls! These shampoos are even more drying on the curls than regular shampoos.

For these extreme curl patterns (at the far end of the curl pattern chart), there are extreme, yet simple, washing routines. Changing your washing routine will make a huge difference to your curls' texture, pattern and definition. First, and most important for your kinky curly pattern, is sulfate-free shampoo. This is a must for your fragile curl pattern. The damaging effects of sulfates on your curls will be greatly magnified compared to what happens to a wavy curl pattern. A wavy curl's cuticle is generally a lot more compact, because that curl doesn't have as many bends. But, as discussed above, kinky curls have a lot of bends, and the cuticle is raised at each bend, where curls are the weakest.

You can either wean yourself off shampoo by switching to a sulfate-free brand and slowly stretching the frequency of your washing and cleansing days or you can go cold turkey. That's the extreme routine suggestion! No shampoo at all. Ideally, you want to get to where you just wet down and condition your curls, until the moisture balance is restored. That's right—no shampoo at all. Even sulfate-free versions have cleansing ingredients that may remove too much moisture from your curl pattern. So if you're game for a shampoo-free routine to get your curls to recover and finally see hair growth, this will help you see a beautiful curl pattern emerge.

Wet your curls as much as you like. Wetting hair down and conditioning with a quality product that has good botanical and hydrating ingredients is not the same as stripping your hair with shampoo. Most of my clients with kinky curly hair are at a three-week-only wash routine. Yes, that's right: they're washing their curls once every three weeks with sulfate-free shampoo. The rest of the time, these curlies just rinse and condition. After my clients have been using this routine for a while, I convert them to a no-shampoo-at-all routine, where they're only co-washing, eliminating shampoo entirely. (Co-washing, you may recall from earlier chapters, is using only conditioner to clean your scalp and moisturize curls when needed.)

Steps to Curl Recovery

These are the steps to follow to bring your curls back to life and turn those curls around.

1. The first step in your curl recovery is clarifying, to remove buildup. The clarifying method has been mentioned a few times throughout *The ABCs*. It's a 1:2 paste made of baking soda and sulfate-free shampoo or conditioner. See the "Washing & Conditioning" chapter (p. 33) for full instructions.

2. Find the best conditioner that provides the moisture you need for your hair. Research curl patterns with your texture online, check reviews, and with a little trial and error, you will find the right one. Choose one that is rich in botanical ingredients and emollients to restore moisture and provide hydration to the cuticle and curls.

3. Avoid conditioners with a lot of oils as main ingredients while you're going through curl recovery; your conditioner will be your staple. Exceptions are products where the oils are water soluble.

4. Be careful of falling into a kinky curly protein treatment kick. Too much protein can actually harden your curls and make them drier.

5. If you're using the right conditioner, you can leave up to 50 percent of the conditioner in your hair, as this curl pattern needs as much moisture as possible left in as a hydrating base.

6. If curls still feel as though they need more moisture, find a leave-in conditioner to layer on top.

7. Follow steps for proper product application as described in the "Styling Your Curls" chapter (the pinch and glide frizz buster method, p. 91, is recommended).

8. Don't be afraid to use gel in your hair. It will act as a cocoon to protect your tender little curls and seal all the benefits of your conditioner(s) in your hair. Use an alcohol-free product, if possible.

9. If you are using a satin bonnet to sleep in, toss it away! Because of the denseness of hair at your scalp, your curl pattern in particular needs as much oxygen as possible to allow your scalp to breathe. All

that those satin bonnets, caps and do-rags do is suffocate the scalp. Read the "Sleeping Curly" chapter to find your curls' best bedtime friend for ways to sleep and protect your curls.

10. Most people with kinky curls have drier scalps. If your scalp flakes, don't worry: in time, your scalp will normalize. Your previous shampooing routine stripped the oils from your hair, so your scalp needs time to create the good natural oils at a new pace in accordance with your new routine. Keep in mind you've been doing a certain routine for years and it's going to take a little time to correct your hair and scalp.

11. Stimulate the scalp when conditioning. Use circular motions with your fingertips everywhere to get the sebaceous glands (which produce the oils your scalp naturally creates) working. If your scalp remains dry, you can try gently massaging *jojoba oil* into the scalp. Jojoba is similar to the consistency of your natural oils created by your scalp's sebaceous glands.

Using Oils for Hydration & Shine

I only have a handful of curlies who tell me they use various oil-laden products on their hair routinely and actually have good curls as a result. When I say handful, I mean fewer than 10. Those with kinky curls seek shine, but don't be discouraged if you don't see it in your hair. Our straighter-haired friends have a smooth hair surface that easily reflects the light, creating shine. Most zigzag kinky curl patterns (aka fractal curls) have next to no visible bends in the hair to reflect light. Don't try to create the illusion of shine by applying oils to your hair. Shine is not a reflection of healthy hair. Slathering your head in butters and oils, if not done properly, will only suffocate and damage your hair and cause more dryness.

However, if you must use oils, choose lightweight ones, and apply only on top of a conditioner that has been left in your hair. Refer to the section about when and how to use oils in the "Product Knowledge" chapter. Curlies with kinky curls are the number one over-users of castor oil. Put it away!

Castor oil should only be 0.7 percent of any formula, so when it's used at full strength directly on the curls, it's very damaging and drying. No matter how many decades your family has been using this method and product, know that it's not good for your curls.

As you move forward in your kinky curly hair journey, you may want to find a way to show a little more curl pattern definition. Highlights are a good option for you. Highlights do not have to be blond or an extreme contrast to your natural color to show definition; consider a toffee or caramel shade, or a copper or red tone. A nice effect is to highlight random tips of your curls. But before you opt for chemical services such as highlights, read the "Color & Highlights" chapter to ensure you find a stylist who will use the proper techniques so your curl pattern stays as healthy as can be.

> ***Note:*** *If you have been using henna products on your curls, you should not have any chemical color services: no highlights, or full or partial colors until all the henna has been grown out. Henna changes the elasticity of the hair and you wouldn't want your hair breaking off now that you are trying to get your curls healthy. In any case, a test strand done before any chemical service to check the curls' integrity is suggested.*

Curl Story

In closing this chapter, I want to share one of my favorite stories with you. I have a client from Jamaica who is in her 60s. Her hair was so dehydrated and damaged when we met: I couldn't even identify her curl pattern. Her curls felt and looked like fine steel wool. She came to me at the end of her rope and almost in tears. She just didn't know what to do with her curls. Her hair was about one inch long, a TWA (Teeny Weeny Afro). Her curls were breaking off in pieces. She had zero curl pattern or definition—just frizz.

This curly didn't know about shampoo or conditioning routines for curly hair. All she knew was that since she had stopped relaxing her hair with chemical straighteners, her hair was not as healthy as she thought it would be. Her scalp was constantly flaking, dry and itchy, and she never noticed any hair growth. The more she washed her hair, the more it would break off and the more her scalp would flake. She was using a very popular dandruff shampoo at the time she came to see me. She was also using oils on her hair in hopes of adding much-needed moisture. Nothing was working.

I spent about 90 minutes with this kinky curly lady. I clarified her hair with a paste of baking soda and sulfate-free shampoo to remove the oil buildup. I then gave her a light protein treatment from my organic line to help restore some elasticity. We spoke about what she had to do moving forward:

- No more regular shampoo; she could use a sulfate-free shampoo, but only occasionally, as needed.
- No more oils, especially castor oil.
- No satin bonnets; she was to sleep with the hair free.
- She needed to find a conditioner her curls liked and leave the product in her hair.
- She could wet down her hair as much as she wished, then condition, condition, condition!

I told her the more often she gave her curls the TLC (Tender Love & Conditioner) they craved, the faster they would recover. She had found me from referrals online and just trusted that I knew what I was talking about because of the reviews and took all my advice to heart. I saw the look on her face as I was going through the curl coaching, and got the sense she was thinking that my advice was almost too simple. At the end of her appointment, she asked whether that was all she had to do. Yes, I said, that's it!

Less than a month later I called to check in with her, and she had turned her curly hair around. She said her hair was no longer breaking and her scalp was not itching and flaking; her curls were coming along much better. Within two years, she had four inches of visible hair growth and a heart-shaped curly hairstyle. I gave her beautiful highlights to provide contrast to her natural color to show off her now defined curl pattern, which we had eventually determined was 4b.

This woman had spent a lifetime searching for her curls, and now that she's found them, she's wearing them proudly. Last time this kinky curly lady came in, she was under the hooded dryer taking selfies! I know she shares with everyone how simply giving up shampoo and just co-washing has changed her curly world! I'm so proud of her and totally amazed at her transition: she stuck to the simple rules I gave her and her curly hair blossomed.

So, kinky curlies, the best advice I can give in a nutshell is to minimize your shampooing frequency, and consider not shampooing at all, but co-washing instead. Provide your curls with lots of TLC, and find *and use* the best conditioner you feel hydrates your hair. Make sure you cleanse and stimulate your scalp well with massages when you co-wash. Throw out that satin cap or just save it to wear when you're cooking with the oils you're now only using in the pan to cook your food and not on your curls. Let your curls and scalp breathe and they will give back to you the most amazing texture, definition and growth!

Chapter 11

Color & Highlights

Just as curly hair requires specific techniques to cut and shape your curls, so are there specific methods used to color and/or highlight your curls. Your hair should be in a healthy state before booking any chemical service. I have turned many clients away after they booked a consultation to discuss color services if I've determined their hair was not healthy enough. Why cause further damage? If your hair is dehydrated and not well on its way to curl recovery, use some of the methods suggested in this guide, and wait before looking to color your hair.

Research your color options online based on your curl pattern and the look you are hoping to achieve. Take pictures to your stylist so together you can make the best color and technique choices for you. Be realistic in your hair color goals. If you have black hair and you want to be blond, keep your expectations reasonable. This particular color change will not happen overnight, or at least not safely in one appointment without compromising the health of your curls.

Curl Story

My 3b kinky curly client with black hair came to me as a newbie a few years ago. Her hair goal was to be blonde. She was a recovering flat-iron junkie and her hair was not at all in a healthy state. I told her she needed to get her hair in better condition before we did any services. I explained that her blonde ambition would not happen overnight without compromising her curl pattern, so we had to proceed slowly. She came back for a trim three months later and her curls were in a much better state. I took her hair a couple of shades lighter at each appointment; in between, she would condition and do treatments at home to keep her hair healthy. It took three appointments, spaced three months apart, to allow her curls time to recover. We achieved the color she wanted safely and her curl pattern remained 100 percent intact—but it took time. So, if you are in the same situation and your stylist of choice says, "Yes, I can do that service for you today," be prepared for extreme damage to your hair texture and curl pattern. More than likely, the damage won't be reversible. Your hair will have to grow out to be healthy again. There are a few curly enigmas out there who can take excessive chemical service abuse and still be okay. But do you really want to take the chance that you're that one in a million?

This Curly Stylist's Experience with Color

As with every other step for curls in this book, I have an opinion on color lines, certain ingredients and how those ingredients affect curly hair. Whether you color your hair at the salon or at home, if you find that your curls are dehydrated and excessively frizzy when your hair is not only dry but when wet as well, your curl pattern is not holding a curl or your scalp feels irritated while color is processing, I suggest you avoid colors with ingredients such as ammonia and PPD (paraphenylenediamine or p-phenylenediamine). PPD is an oxidative ingredient used in hair colorants that makes it so the color can penetrate and process for permanent hair color change, especially for gray coverage. Ammonia has been used for decades in color formulas for the same reasons.

I am not a scientist, but what I have noticed over the years, comparing different color lines, is that these two ingredients can be very drying on all types of curls, cause irritation to the scalp and affect the curl pattern and shine. Research shows that in many cases, these ingredients dry out the hair and strip it of its natural health (elasticity) and shine. When I started using color lines with no PPD (or just very low concentrations) and no ammonia, my clients' hair became much healthier and shinier, and had better curl retention. Also, 99 percent of my clients noticed the products without these two ingredients did not irritate the scalp. The one percent who experience hypersensitivity have severe allergies to everything from foods to cosmetics, so even the gentlest color formulas irritate their scalp.

Curlies who came to me for color service from high-end salons that use the best-known professional brands noticed immediately that there was no irritation to their scalp and no chemical odors. Within a few applications, they see hair that is less frizzy, and has better curl retention, a defined curl pattern and more shine. Elasticity, you now know, contributes to the hair's ability to hold a curl. Compromising the elasticity by using ingredients that strip the hair is not beneficial in keeping that curl pattern healthy. When seeking a color service, find out what color lines the salon uses and whether there are PPD- and ammonia-free options.

For the Curly Who Loves Black-Colored Hair

So, black beauty, when you dye your hair that lovely shade you favor so much, you must keep in mind that should you decide to get highlights, or maybe go a lighter shade of brown, it is very difficult to penetrate black dyes. The pigments used in black dyes are so concentrated to achieve that degree of darkness, it's a difficult color to change without using high levels of peroxide to lift you part of the way safely to the shade you may want. In the future, if you choose a level 5 (almost all color lines will have a number on the box), which is considered dark or darkest brown, your hair will still appear close to black. Level 5 is a lot easier to work with for coloring and lifting to lighter shades, or providing highlighting services, than level 1 black.

Communication

Always, *always* be honest with your hairstylist about your hair history. Tell your stylist what products, dyes or hennas you have used and for how long. Should you want a color change or highlights, the stylist will then know what steps to take and tell you the results to expect. Don't think that because it's been maybe six months to two or more years ago since you've dyed your hair that it doesn't make a difference. It does. The color you'll be getting will process completely differently near the roots than on the ends of previously colored hair. If you want the best results possible, be truthful, even if you're embarrassed because you did a bad at-home color. This will help eliminate the unknown for your stylist and therefore help avoid poor color results.

Prepping for Hair Color Service

Whether you have a sensitive scalp and reactions to hair dye or not, always make sure hair is not freshly washed (maybe even three days since your last wash) so that the scalp can create natural oils to buffer the effects of the dye during processing. Never brush your hair before a color service, as dye may cause irritation during the application and processing if you scratch the scalp with the brush bristles.

Highlight Strand Test

Stylists can offer a strand test to check for allergic reactions, the integrity of your curls when bleach is applied, and how light your hair can go to get to your target shade with one service.

There are two types of tests: one involves snipping a small lock from somewhere at the back lower part of your head a couple of inches up from the base hairline; the other strand test is done right on your curly head. In either case, highlight formula is applied to the lock of hair, then rinsed off. Keep in mind that highlighting a snipped-off lock won't test for allergic reactions, but it can show how light the hair will go and how long it will take to process.

If the strand test has been done to a lock of hair on your head, wait a week or two to see what the color result is after washing, conditioning and styling a couple of times. You can have the strand cut off or dyed back to your natural color should you decide the color service is something you no longer wish to pursue.

Usually this service will have a charge, but it could save you from a mistake that could take years to rectify, depending on the length of your curls. This is your hair, your curls, your crowning glory and it's worth the investment, not only of the fee for the test, but of time and patience when thinking about a chemical service. The only thing I want you to be impatient about is changing your routine and recovering your curls. Be slow to make chemical-service decisions!

Do-It-Yourself Color

Demi-permanent and permanent colors have active ingredients that, when applied to your hair, raise the cuticles to deposit color. Curls become more fragile during a chemical service. You should never rake fingers or comb hair color through your hair when you apply color or at any time while the color is processing. Pulling or tugging singly or combined will damage the curl pattern. If you are doing a full color, scrunch the product into the hair after applying color with a root touch-up color brush to effectively cover your roots and your hair strands. Don't be frugal with your color either. If you need two boxes to coat the hair to save the stress from pulling and spreading product through, use two boxes! If possible, leave this service to a professional stylist.

Keep in mind that curls, and especially dry, porous curly hair or very fine hair, will almost always go one or two shades darker than the box indicates. These hair types will soak up the pigment in the dyes, thus processing a darker color.

Root Touch-Ups

Apply your dye only to your roots and try not to overlap the color down the strand where the demarcation line is (where the previously colored hair starts and the new growth you are coloring meet). Fewer chemicals on the previously colored hair is best to preserve the integrity of your hair. When processing time is done, apply a little warm water to the hair and imagine the color you applied to your roots is now a shampoo. **Gently emulsify** the color shampoo on the roots, then scrunch hair from the ends up to the roots. This action will freshen up the ends without over-processing. Don't rush the emulsifying process. Continue to shampoo in the color for at least three minutes, as it will further encourage the color to penetrate the whole hair shaft. After coloring, or any other chemical service, always seal hair with a good conditioner or treatment to restore moisture balance.

Curly Color Tip

To give a true colour freshening to your ends, mix up a couple of ounces of color with the peroxide developer (depending how long and thick your hair is), and dilute the mixture with half the amount of the total liquid you have mixed using distilled water. So, if you have mixed 2 ounces total of permanent color, add 1 ounce of distilled water and apply to your hair from the end of where the root touch-up ends to the ends of your hair when it's 5 minutes from the end of your root color processing time. Scrunch the color mixture into the hair. Follow the steps above from "Gently emulsify."

Color Too Dark?

If you've applied a color that is a little too dark, try using a shampoo cocktail consisting of 2 ounces 20 volume peroxide, 1 ounce shampoo and 1 ounce warm water; apply to wet hair and allow the solution to rest on your hair. Lifting the color can be as quick as 30 seconds to a couple of minutes maximum, so be sure to monitor the color change. Rinse out, cleanse and condition. You may need to see a professional who is experienced in color correction if you are not successful yourself.

Gray Options

Now, I love silver highlights and think being fully natural is great, but some curlies (both men and women) prefer full-coverage color for the silver babies. If you just have a few gray strands, you can opt for what I call the strand-by-strand color method. If you like your natural color but don't like the few grays you have, apply a permanent, demi-permanent or semi-permanent color matching your hair color to the grays strand by strand. Or, if you only have some patches of gray at the temples or by the ears (which seems to be where the grays are more predominant as we age), simply apply color to those areas only. There is no need to cover your whole head with chemicals for just a little gray. Semi-permanent will wash out more quickly than demi-permanent, while permanent color does not wash away.

Resistant Gray Hair

You can alter the amount of developer mixed with permanent color to make a formula richer in pigment for those resistant grays that just won't cover. For example, if the color you use is to be mixed 1:1 ratio (one part color to one part peroxide), adjust the formula so it's 1 ounce color mixed with ¾ ounce 20 volume cream peroxide. Always use 20 volume peroxide for permanent color formulas; anything lower (like a 10 volume) will not raise the cuticle enough to make that permanent color change or cover grays.

> **Note:** *Make sure you go to a professional stylist with the appropriate training for chemical services. If your budget and time don't allow, try to buy professional colors from professional beauty suppliers. Find a color line that is PPD- and/or ammonia-free, which is less damaging to your hair.*

A Few Grays to Cover

If you have only a little gray to cover, highlights or lowlights can be added to blend in with the grays to soften them. Highlights don't need to be blond; you can go a few shades lighter than your natural tone or darker to break up the concentration of gray hair, so the grays won't stand out so much.

Don't worry if you're a "gray plucker." There is no scientific evidence to support the notion that when you pull one gray hair, 10 grow back!

Quick Gray-Fix Touch-Ups

Curly hair hides grays well, but it's the areas around the face that are troublesome and make it hard for some clients to last six weeks between color or root touch-up services. If this is the case with you, do what I call a "face frame color touch-up"—a mini-color service applied to where the grays show more quickly. You can more than likely do one or two face frames before you have to do a full root touch-up. It saves you time and money, and you and your scalp are exposed to fewer chemicals. If you try to stretch the full root touch-up past two quick fixes, you may find it hard to cover the grays and regrowth properly. A touch-up can also include a part line, too, if you have visible gray there. Apply color on the part line and one section over on each side of the part to allow for when your hair falls differently when styling your hair.

Reducing the Frequency of Root Touch-Up Applications

If you only have a few visible grays after a couple of weeks, opt for one of the many dry color sticks, hair powder or hair mascara for temporary gray coverage solutions to stretch your color service and have fewer chemicals on your scalp as often. I've also found that water-resistant eye shadows (if you can find the right shade) will work well, too! Just apply to roots or grays as you would a color stick, but use a makeup applicator brush. See

Temporary Wash-to-Wash Solutions in the next chapter, "Gray & Color Transitioning," for available products.

Henna

Out of all the clients I have met, only one client has the perfect unaffected curl using henna. She uses the true henna paste with no chemicals added. The others curlies are using box dyes marked as "henna" from the health food store; their curls are dry, brittle and brassy as a result. Cosmetologists are taught that henna affects the elasticity of the hair and is therefore damaging. If a client is using henna and comes in for a chemical service, we're told we must do a strand test, as the hair may break off and suffer extreme, if not irreparable, damage when combined with another chemical service. It's therefore essential that you're honest with your stylist if you've been using henna at home and have now decided to get professional color services done, so your stylist can use appropriate test strands if necessary before your service to check the integrity of your curls.

Highlights/Lowlights

These are wonderful techniques. When done correctly, you are exposing your scalp to minimal chemicals. They can also enhance your curl and add definition to the tighter kinky curly 3 to 4 hair patterns. When seeking a stylist to provide this service, choose one who does not use foils. Some high-end salons will use special highlight paper or foam strips. At my studio, I use a unique technique utilizing a paper that does not accelerate the process, as do foils. The end result is healthy curls with minimal damage and less compromise to the curl pattern.

Why avoid foil highlights? When the bleach and developer are combined and trapped between the foils, a chemical reaction is created: The cuticle is blasted open by the heat produced in these foil packets where the hair has been pressed straight when the bleach was applied. This stretches out the curl, and that contributes to the highlighted pieces taking on a looser curl pattern than the curls that were not highlighted. If you were to touch a foil pocket while your hair is processing, you would feel the heat. In some cases, the foil pouch puffs up as the chemical reaction occurs. Using foil as an accelerator pushes this process to the extreme by literally cooking the hair.

Balayage is a French technique whereby bleach is lightly stroked on the hair in a random fashion and is left to process under a cap, not trapped within foil. This is a much better way to achieve highlights, but is more suitable for a looser curl pattern as opposed to a tighter one, as it may not provide even coverage along kinky curly strands.

Why Do Salons Use Foil for Highlights?

Stylists at salons are locked into a technique created decades ago but still taught today. In a salon, foil is easily accessible and most stylists are educated in its applications. Salons allow a certain amount of time for highlight services and foil allows for quick processing. Although alternative highlight papers and foam highlight strips have been developed and available for years, in most cases, using these papers will take longer for the hair to process, because they do not create the heat foil does. Also, paper and foam cost much more than aluminum foil, which is inexpensive and easily accessible. Using foil is a time- and money-saving product for salons.

But using foil doesn't take into consideration your hair's health. If choosing to highlight your hair, your goal as a curly will be to find a stylist who offers an alternative to foil highlights. The service may be a little more expensive when special techniques are used, but it's well worth the investment to protect your curly pattern.

Lowlights, whether done with paper or foam, will take the same time to do as foil, since these color formulas don't need heat to process. However, if your hair is very resistant (compact cuticle that needs heat to raise it) or you want a lighter shade that needs a little extra boost, heat from a hooded dryer will be needed to activate the developer and bleach.

Curl Stories

Shortly after I graduated from Avola College for Cosmetology, I went to visit my former teacher, Mrs. Armstrong. While I was there, I went to another part of the school to get my highlights done by a senior student. He applied them perfectly. Shortly after the processing began, the supervising teacher came to watch as the student tested a strand to see if my hair was light enough. As he reached for the aluminum foil with a towel in his hand to rub away the bleach to check whether the color was processed, my gut told me this was the wrong thing to do. All of a sudden it clicked in what was going to happen. I told the teacher he was going to ruin the curl in my bangs if he rubbed the bleach off to test with that towel. It was too late. He had already rubbed the curl out of my hair! It only took seconds and it was done.

The teacher said my comment was ridiculous. He worked for decades at many high-end salons, so what could I, as a younger, newer stylist, possibly have to offer in the way of knowledge except to point to the long straggly bang left hanging from the foil? After my hair was washed and styled, the only thing ridiculous was my straight hair where the student rubbed the bleach off to do a test strand. I learned firsthand when working with chemicals why it is so important to be gentle with hair when it is processing. No testing strands by rubbing, brushing, combing or finger raking product through the hair while being chemically processed. These actions compromise the curl pattern!

Years ago, I was so shocked to see a stylist tap a flat iron against a client's highlight foil packets to force the process to move along by applying heat. The poor little curls were a mess as a result! No or minimal heat is best during processing, if possible, and no tapping the foil packet with a flat iron!

The moral of these curly stories? Save the foil for cooking food, not your curls!

Always Remember!

As a client, make sure you follow your instincts when you're in the stylist's chair and care. You know your curls better than anyone, especially more than the stylist you may have only met three minutes earlier at your first appointment. Even if you have seen the same stylist several times before, he or she is still getting to know your hair. Yes, stylists are educated in the care of hair, but just as there are good and not so good mechanics, plumbers and nail technicians, there are stylists who are not as good as others or trained in the techniques you may want.

Do research beforehand, call the salon and check reviews from other clients who have been to that stylist. If ever you sense that a service is not going the way you think it should, feel the processing time is too long, have an irritated scalp or see your stylist heading out for a smoke when you think your processing is done, say something. Don't just allow the processing to continue. You are the client, and as much as we like to put faith in the training and ability of our stylists, sometimes you have to speak up and not just freeze in the stylist's chair when your gut tells you something may not be right!

Chapter 12

Gray & Color Transitioning

You've been dying to stop dyeing your hair for years and have decided it's time to get off the color wagon. It's a decision you could be making for many reasons. You may not want to commit to coloring your hair any longer because of the time, effort or money spent on color services. Maybe you want a healthier lifestyle and want to be free of the bondage of permanent color touch-ups and chemicals on your scalp! You may not even be coloring your hair to cover grays and have decided you want to grow in your own natural hair color. You'll most likely now have to deal with the downside of the color transition, especially if stopping covering grays or there's a big difference between the color of your dyed hair and natural shade: the skunk line, which is the strong band, or demarcation line, where the natural hair color and dyed color meet. There are, however, some options to help as you grow out the dyed hair.

Quit Color Cold Turkey

- Persevere and live with the skunk line as your natural hair grows in. Get frequent trims to close the gap between your colored hair and the natural hair coming in at the root. Hair grows at a rate of about six inches a year (½ inch every two months), so it could take a little time to grow out, depending on your hair length.

Dark Hair Transition

- If you are growing out hair that is dyed a darker color than your natural shade, consider semi-permanent or demi-permanent hair color formulas applied to the regrowth until the permanent hair color has been trimmed off.
- Semi-permanent colors don't use developers or peroxide to process the color, so you can't lift hair color to a lighter shade, and they last 6 to12 washes. Demi-permanent formulas use a low level of peroxide and last from 12 to 24 washes.
- Semi-permanent colors may not provide total coverage on your natural hair and may result in a tonal change that is translucent, because it doesn't contain the amount of peroxide that permanent colors do.
- How long semi-permanent or demi-permanent colors last will depend on how well your hair holds color and how often you wash your hair.
- Trim hair every three months or so to remove the permanently colored ends; closing the gap between your natural hair and dyed ends takes time, depending on the length of your hair.
- Once you have trimmed off all the permanent-colored ends, you'll be able to stop with the temporary color process, so the last color you do will fade and you can sport your natural color.

  Note: *If you have really resistant hair that doesn't color easily, even when you use permanent color, using temporary color may not be an option for you, because of the lower peroxide levels in* *these formulas. A color patch test done by your hairstylist will show how well the color will hold on your hair.*

Light Hair / Blond Transition

- If you have been dyeing your hair blond or a high lift shade, you may opt for highlights on your regrowth to gradually grow in your natural hair color. Highlights are permanent and can help break the stark contrast of the demarcation line as you grow out your blond ends.
- If you are transitioning to gray from hair that was dyed blond, you could choose to do lowlights in a demi-permanent lighter brown color (lowlights in too dark a tone will make you look stripy). The lowlights will add a little dimension to your roots and down the previously colored ends to help with the stark look of your natural gray hair growing in.
- You can apply both highlights and lowlights from roots to ends until you grow in your natural color. Both will help break up the demarcation line to make the color transition easier for you to live with.
- Get a trim every three months or so to close the gap between the colored blond ends and the natural hair growth.

"My Natural Gray Color Is Boring and Blah!"

- You can add highlights (which are permanent), or semi-permanent or demi-permanent lowlights if you don't want to commit to a permanent color that will fade out.
- Both these color techniques are applied away from the scalp, so chemicals are not processing on your skin, making them healthier color options.
- Highlights will nicely brighten up the gray monotone, while the lightness provided by the highlights will give the illusion of more volume to the hair.
- Applying lowlights will add dimension and depth to your gray tone. Lowlights will give the illusion of less volume to your hair.

- Both highlights and lowlights can be done as frequently as every few months or, for a very low-commitment color service, just once or twice a year and can give you the lift you need to your base color.

Growing Out Permanent Color to Grow In Your Natural Color

- When growing out permanent color to return to your natural color (if you are not transitioning to gray), you can apply an all-over permanent hair color that matches your natural color at the roots.
- Pick a color as close to your natural one as possible. Over time, if the processed hair growing out turns a little brassy or does not match as well with your natural color growing in, you can have toners applied to neutralize those unwanted tones as you grow out the permanent color. Toners are gentle, non-permanent colors that gradually fade out and use very low developers to process, even lower than those in demi-permanent colors.

Color Pigment Shampoos and Conditioners

- For hair that is less resistant and accepts color easily, an at-home option is to use color pigment hair shampoos or conditioners, available at select stores and beauty supply outlets.
- Available in an assortment of basic colors, these shampoos and conditioners have color-rich pigments added to their formulas that add tones to the hair or neutralize unwanted tones.
- Their processing time is short and they do not use any developers or peroxide, so they are not permanent colors.
- Color pigment shampoos and conditions usually last from wash to wash; some single applications can last a week or more. How long the color lasts depends on the concentration of the pigment in the product, how resistant your hair is to cover and how often you wash your hair.

Note: If your hair is very dry or brittle, it will tend to absorb the pigment to the max and in some cases may not rinse out. A test strand will show you how well the product will work for you—make sure you follow the product's directions.

Temporary Wash-to-Wash Solutions

These products are ideal for gray coverage or to help cover the roots as you grow out your permanent color. You can find most of these products at either the drugstore or beauty supply outlet. Most come in a variety of shades to blend with your hair color.

- Hard color sticks are wax-based crayons. Follow the product instructions, but generally, the color stick should be wet when using and applied to wet hair, then blended in with your finger if you get it on your skin, which removes it from the skin and not the hair you have just applied it to.
- Pigment color spray or powder is either sprayed or sprinkled on your hair; these can make hair a little stiff or sticky.
- Color hair markers (similar to a regular marker you would write with) will cover the hair well, but I find they'll cause the hair to become dry and coarse over time.
- Liquid hair mascara comes in an applicator bottle similar to the mascara you use for your eyelashes. The applicator may be a fine comb or sponge tip. These products cover well but can leave the hair sticky.
- Compact pressed-powder hair makeup comes with an applicator brush similar to what you would use to apply eye shadow and leaves a very soft, natural feel to the hair you are covering.

These temporary wash-to-wash solutions don't usually come off during sports or when your hair gets wet from a little rain or sweat from a workout. The cost for these products ranges from around $8 (wax color stick) to $45 (compact hair powders and sprays).

Curly Tip

If you can find a water-resistant eye shadow to match your hair color, you can use that with an eye shadow applicator brush to cover your roots as well. It's a much more economical alternative to the more expensive compact color powders for hair, which can cost up to $45.

I have helped quite a few clients color transition to natural. It's truly all in the way you approach this process. Don't feel aged because of the gray hair. You will have to make sure you provide a balance; don't let the way you carry yourself age you. Just because you are going to go natural with your hair color doesn't mean you shouldn't dress nicely (even if casual), wear a little lipstick, accessorize your outfits and, most importantly, have a good wavy or curly cut and style!

Hair is a big part of the image we project. If you're a curly who has struggled with the curly side your whole life, I'm sure this color transition decision will come with its own set of challenges. Okay, so you'll have roots growing out—just make sure the rest of your package is put together and you'll get through the color transition just fine.

You have to be ready for the change. It would be nice to have family and friends support your decision, too. It's not always the case, though. But, at the end of the day, you're the boss of you and it's your decision to make! If you've already overcome your curl rehab, learned your ABCs and are now rocking your curls, you've already won most of the battle. With a little time and effort, you'll be amazed at how great you'll look with your combo natural color grown in and naturally curly hair!

Chapter 13

Haircuts: Dry vs. Wet & Other Techniques

Regardless of the curl pattern you have, you know curly hair reacts much differently than straight hair in all areas of washing, styling and, of course, cutting. You can't use the same methods for cutting curls as you would for straight hair. The standard wet cut at a regular salon would be great if you are a curly who will always straighten your hair. However, when traditionally trained stylists use the comb to pull wet hair smooth to one length to cut it, that technique doesn't take into consideration the different curl patterns or spring factor. The end result is an uneven shape and style. You will see visible "shelves and ledges" where your curl pattern may be tighter at the crown, or you may end up with longer sides not blended with the length at the back where your hair may not be as curly as the sides. Even worse, you could have bangs that will bounce all the way up to the top of your forehead because the shrinkage of your curlier bangs were not taken into consideration when cut with the straight-hair approach.

A stylist (whether curly trained or not) should not razor-cut your curls or use texturizing techniques (such as point cutting or thinning shears) to remove weight or bulk from your hair. Random texturizing will not achieve the result you're looking for. If you go to a stylist and say, "I feel my hair is heavy right here," and point to a specific area, the stylist will texturize or thin out that area randomly, without targeting the growth pattern, and the styling technique will garner less than satisfying curly results. A stylist properly trained in curly hair will be able to deal with the weight issues using the appropriate techniques for your hair.

A big consideration for cutting curls is the shrinkage factor. Did you know that certain curl patterns can stretch 75 percent or more when wet? That means cutting one inch of curl when it's wet translates into 1¾ inches when dried. A traditionally trained stylist who may not be familiar with what the shrinkage is for each curl pattern could take off a lot of length without realizing it. I'm not saying every stylist has to be certified to deal with curls. However, you need to find one who understands the uniqueness of curly hair and how to take into consideration the spring factor when providing services. If you don't know a traditionally trained stylist who knows how to deal with curls, it's time to look for a curly hair expert.

If you are new to the curly world and are interested in going to a curl expert, the best way to maximize your experience and get the best curly bang for your buck is to make sure your hair is in the best condition possible. Follow the routines you have learned in *The ABCs* to get your curls into curl recovery. Once you've gotten the ABCs down and you're ready for your first curly cut, it's time to decide which curly cutting technique is best for you: there are a variety available today. Below I cover a few of the most common and explain how they differ, but do your research and choose which technique is the most suitable for you.

Dry Cuts

The dry cutting technique is a great cutting style that deals with shape. Curls are cut either curl by curl or in small subsections to create the desired shape. Minimal tension is applied when the curls are cut so there is a visual balance obtained according to how your curls fall. Done properly, a dry cut will allow hair to be styled both curly and straight. However, you must go to your curly stylist with your hair in its natural curly state with your hair washed and styled. When booking your appointment, check with the stylist about whether you should use styling products or not. If hair is in its natural curly state, your stylist can accurately assess your curl pattern and provide the best cutting techniques for your curls.

DON'T go to your appointment with:

- a scrunchy in your hair
- hair sprayed back with product
- hair pinned up or bobby pinned
- curls in a ponytail
- hair blow-dried, flat-ironed or finger-coiled

Any of the above will make it really difficult to dry cut your hair, because the stylist won't be able to see your proper curl pattern. As a result, some stylists will first wash and condition your hair to get your curls in their natural state. You may be charged extra for the service if your hair needs to be detangled. A trim and reshaping is required every six to eight weeks to maintain short hairstyles and every three to six months for medium and longer styles to refresh the ends.

Tunnel (aka Channel or Undercutting) Technique

This particular method is done on wet hair. Some stylists target random sections (tunnel, or channel, cutting) to remove weight from your hair. Hair is either cut close to or shaved to the scalp, while the longer hair conceals the shaved portions. This technique may be used all over the head in varying degrees to remove weight and bulk from the curls. This cutting method requires commitment by the client. As the hair grows out, there will be random sprouts of hair popping out at the scalp. This technique can encourage curls thanks to the weight being removed. If you have a lot of hair and find it overwhelming to manage and style, removing a lot of weight will make the styling process easier. You would need this cut approximately every two to four months, depending on how quickly your hair grows and "sprouting" appears from the shaved portion's growth protruding from the root.

Wet Curly Cut

This cutting technique should be done by a curly stylist who really knows curls and will account for the shrinkage after your hair is dried. This type of cut deals with shape and areas of weight, and will even encourage curl, in some cases. Following a dry cut with a wet cut is sometimes suggested for curlies who swing both ways: those who like to style their hair both straight and curly. A stylist who knows how to cut curly hair wet will use minimal tension when cutting different sections, noting the curl patterns to allow for the hair's spring factor. How often this cut is required depends on the length of hair you wish to maintain. Anywhere from six to eight weeks for a short style to three to six months for those who want to let their hair grow or just keep the length with a follow-up cut, trim or reshaping.

Blow-Dry/Flat-Iron Cutting Technique

I'm including this method, since it's available and known as a *curly* cutting technique. This cut, though done on dry hair, will actually mirror the results of a traditional wet cut done for straight hair. This technique is for **curlies who will always be wearing their hair straight** and doesn't take into consideration the different curl patterns you may have on your head. For this *curly* cut, the hair is washed, blow-dried and then flat-ironed. The resulting straight hair (which is not at all a reflection of your curl pattern) is then cut into the desired shape.

I say this cut is for a curly who will always want to be styled straight because if you have a few different curl patterns on your head (like kinky curls at the crown and looser curls everywhere else), you will end up with a lovely mushroom-shaped shelf at the back if you wear your hair curly, or your sides will not blend with your back. I have seen clients many times with this result after having gone to get this cut. The clients loved their hair when they left the salon, but when they washed their hair to go curly, they found it was a misshapen mess, taking anywhere from two to three years to grow out, depending on the starting length of their hair.

Correcting this cut often involves a big chop, if the curly doesn't want to wait for the shelf at the back to grow out. I personally don't ever recommend this cut for any curl pattern. But, to be objective, if there were one curly hair type that this technique could work on, it's the wavy curl who has a uniform curl pattern everywhere. But keep in mind, one flat-iron service can do at least a month's worth of damage to your hair. Your curls get a little angry and hold a grudge when straightened by a flat iron. That means it may take up to one month for the curl to come back to what it was before this flat-iron curly cutting service. So your stylist is actually damaging your curls to cut it. I don't think this is a very proactive curly cutting technique if you want to do what is best for your curls' health or shape.

Styling Tools to Avoid

If a stylist is coming at your hair with texturizing shears (thin or thick) with teeth spaced close together or far apart, that should have your curly head heading for the hills. The result of using texturizers on curls is sprouts of choppy, random pieces sticking out everywhere when your hair is dry. This leads to frizz and takes a long time to grow out. Razor-cuts can also leave straggly ends on curly hair, so you should make sure your stylist does not use any of these tools to cut your curls!

Chapter 14

Finding a Curl Expert
(Preparing for Your Appointment)

Finding a curl expert who is right for you could take some time and effort. The first step is to work on your routine according to *The ABCs* for one to two months (a little longer if you were a flat-iron junkie) to allow your curls to recover before booking an appointment. Waiting will give needed time for your hair's elasticity to recover, if you haven't pushed your curls past the point of no curl return: where you have damaged the cuticles using poor washing or conditioning practices, chemical or heat services, or a combination of any of these so much that the elasticity can't be restored. In most cases, when curls are being conditioned properly and are not being stripped by sulfates or being blow-dried or flat-ironed, they will recover. Once you think your curl pattern is back as much as it can be, then book your appointment. The curly stylist can then see what she or he is working with. The last thing you want is to rush to find a curly stylist, get two inches cut off before your hair has recovered its elasticity and then discover that the two inches cut off a month ago is now four inches as the elasticity returns, thanks to completing your curl recovery with your new-found routines.

The exception to the wait time is curlies using chemical relaxers or straighteners. When the hair's bonds have been totally broken with relaxers and straightening systems, they will not come back. The washing practices and ABCs' rules implemented into your routine will benefit new growth at the root. As you move forward with your curly journey, it will be up to you and your curls whether you do a big chop (remove all the straight ends that no longer have a curl pattern) or take off little bits at a time while using protective styling methods. You may get tired of trying to style the flat ends to blend with the new root growth or hiding the great curly roots with scarves until your ends are cut off. It can be a long process, depending on the starting length of your hair.

As suggested, seeking a stylist would be most beneficial after curl recovery. Don't rush into booking your appointment with a curly hair expert without first doing research. You're investing in your hair, and the stylist you hope to find will help you with your curls face to face. Generally, curly stylists who have received special training with curls will cost more than a regular hair stylist. As explained in Chapter 13, "Haircuts: Dry vs. Wet & Other Techniques," there are various cutting techniques, so research which one you think will be best for your curls and look for a stylist trained in that technique.

Here are steps to help you find the best salon and stylist for your curls.

Google "curly hair salons or stylist" (usually Google will bring up a listing of those geographically closest to you). From that list, Google the name of the salon or stylist. Check online for reviews. Call the salon and ask about the cutting techniques and who's certified to cut curly hair.

Consider the following:

- how long the stylist has been trained or certified
- what the cost is for a cut
- what's included with the service
- whether there are junior and senior stylists available and what the differences in cost and services are
- if there is a consultation fee and how long the consultation is
- book a consultation if you feel you need to meet the stylist to discuss services and determine if you are a fit

Before meeting the stylist, make notes of things that are important to you. Keep your points brief; don't use the time with the curly stylist speaking of all the things you and your curls have been through from the beginning of time. You want to focus on where your hair is now, not what it was 20 years ago. These points will assist your stylist:

1. Find pictures on the Internet of shapes you like. Don't bring pictures with curly hair patterns and textures completely different from yours and say, "I want that" or "Wish my hair could do that." Look at realistic shapes, curl patterns specific to yours, and styles according to your curl pattern and current hair length or where you want your length to be.
2. Write down all the things you didn't like about your previous haircuts.
3. Know where your curl patterns differ and point them out; for example, tighter curls at the crown or looser ones at the sides by your ears. Also, identify the areas in which you may experience more dryness.
4. If you are having chemical services done, explain to your curly stylist how your hair reacts to color or highlights. Does your hair process quickly or slowly? Does your hair pull a lot of red when you have had your hair colored, and you hate red? Does your scalp get irritated when you get color done? All this information, which I call "hair history," is relevant and will help your stylist understand your hair.

5. Know your styling goals. Do you want to grow your hair long or keep it a little shorter so it's at shoulder length, because you need to be able to pull it back? Are you looking for layers? Do you like a round shape or more elongated? Do you want more volume or less in your curly style? Do you have a lot of time to spend on your hair or need quick styling?

6. If the stylist is trained in various curly cutting techniques and you know which one you would like, make sure to specify.

7. Once you've expressed your points, and hopefully there have been comments back, let the curly hair expert make suggestions and see how in line they are with your goals. If in doubt, question. You may be nervous and feel some anxiety, which is natural. But a bad vibe and not feeling you're connecting with the stylist is another thing altogether. If you feel the curly stylist is not for you, whether this was a consultation or not, don't feel bad if you do not want to go through with the appointment. This is your hair. You have to feel you have made the right decision and chosen the right curly hair stylist.

Most stylists will do a consultation at the time of service, but if you decide to book a consultation alone and no cutting service, be prepared to pay $20 and up. It will be worth the investment, though, to find the right fit for you and your curls. Some of the points I've asked you to make note of above will in most cases be questions your curly hair expert will ask you at your appointment, so be proactive and be prepared with brief notes.

Charges for curly haircuts are usually based on hair length, but could be a flat rate for any length. If booking a coaching session, which involves teaching you all you need to know about taking care of your curls, be prepared to pay $100 to $250, or even more, depending on how much time the service takes and what credentials the curly stylist has. A lot goes into teaching a new curly hair client. I've had coaching sessions that included treatments and styling that lasted for three hours. That's a lot of time needed to help a curly client, and that's why the services will be more expensive than a regular haircut.

Since you have invested in *The ABCs*, you may not need to book a curl coaching session. I'm not saying the stylist can't teach you more than what's contained here, but you will know a lot already. That said, we learn from everyone in this curly world, so everyone you meet will contribute to your curly knowledge. But people learn in different ways, so even after reading this book, you may want a one-on-one session to help guide you with your curls.

When you find the right stylist, your curly life will change drastically. Some curly hair stylists will teach you little steps at each appointment; others will offer a total curly revamp and rock your world from the first appointment. Either way, take your time finding the right stylist. It's just like finding the right doctor, dentist, manicurist or eyebrow-shaping technician. This is your hair, your waves, your curls. When it's cut, it's done. So, you really have to take control of your hair and find the best person to help you get what you want for your curly hair goals.

Preparing for Your First Appointment

Call the salon a few days before your appointment and ask how they prefer you have your curls when you come in. If you have already begun your curl rehab, as I've strongly recommended, just make sure your hair is washed, styled and *completely* dry, with minimal product so your curl pattern is visible. Do not wear headbands, scrunchies, twists or braids, and do not blow-dry or flat-iron your hair for your first curly appointment. The stylist has to see your curls where the hair actually rests in its natural curly state to cut your curls properly.

Remove the element of surprise by arriving with dry, styled curly hair. Wash and style your hair the night before, or a full day before if your hair takes a long time to dry. Sleep with one of the protective styling methods suggested in "Sleeping Curly." Wake up the next morning, fluff and refresh your curls with a curl refresher or light mist of water, and get ready for your appointment. Again, most importantly, curls should be fully dry prior to a curly cut.

If your hair is very dehydrated, the stylist may suggest a treatment before the cut, followed by a wash and style, to make sure you get the best results. I don't think a treatment would be suggested if it was not needed. Do question it, though, if you feel that you don't need it. Every extra service, and the more time the curly stylist spends on your hair, will add to the final price. A base cut price that needs a pre-service, such as a treatment, will cost more.

Know that only so much can be accomplished in one appointment—especially if you have frayed and broken hair at different lengths from neglect or curl abuse, or have not had a cut for years out of curly fear. Have realistic expectations. A stylist may even see your fear and anxiousness and suggest just a slight cleanup or trim to freshen all the ends at your first appointment. This may not give the best shape, but it will help establish trust. Communication is key, so discuss your curly fears during your pre-cut consultation.

If you jumped to book your appointment before finishing curl rehab, your curls may look great when you leave the salon, but as your hair recalls its past abuse, it will return to the old, dry, frizzy habits before the day is done. Another scenario is your hair looks absolutely fantastic: lasts for days, curls are great. Then you wash your curls and try to recreate the style and it doesn't look the same. Ask yourself these questions:

1. Are you using the same products the stylist did?
2. Did you apply the products the same way?
3. Did you dry your hair the same way as at the salon?

Answer no to even just one of those questions and there's your reason why. To recreate a style, in most cases you have to recreate the steps. Don't be so quick to be disappointed with the results. If, however, you did everything the same way as at the salon, call the stylist to figure out where you may have gone wrong. You're building a relationship with the stylist. Curly hair experts are in that field not only because they love hair, but love curly hair and love helping the curly person. It's such a special niche. If you're at all disappointed in a service, follow up with any concerns—don't be quick to break up with your first curly date!

Before your appointment, consider your curls' length and bounce. If in doubt about how much length you wish to cut off, ask the stylist to leave your hair a bit longer, especially if taking off a lot of inches. By removing length, you are removing weight that holds your curls down and elongates them; your curls may bounce up quite a bit shorter. It's better to go a little on the long side than to take off too much length.

Although I'm trained in various curl-cutting methods, 9 times out of 10 I do a dry cut for new curly clients. That way, the client can see how much length is lost when the hair is in its natural curly state. I can target the very dry strands, for example, that may have altered the curl pattern from previous highlighting or color services that would not show if I cut the hair when wet. As my clients continue along their curl journey and want to deal with weighty areas or encourage more curl through alternative cutting methods, I will introduce those services at a later date.

There are various terms for curl cuts. Trims and "dusting" refer to cleaning up the ends. If unsure of the terms used at the salon, simply inquire. There are no silly questions in the curly world. Make sure to keep your curly ends fresh. If you wait too long between cuts, the ends will fray and you won't see much growth happening. On average, a curly cut is every two to six months. Do weekly or biweekly treatments and you may be able to stretch your curly cuts to six-month intervals. The two-month periods or less are for short curly cuts that need more frequent attention to keep their shape.

So, now you're on your way. You know how to approach your first appointment with a curly stylist. Don't forget to take your before and after selfies at your first curly appointment! You'll need them to add to the curly rehab collection you've started.

Chapter 15

Curl Bits

Ever wonder why your curls are behaving a certain way, unaware that it may be something in your routine that could be causing an unfavorable curly side effect? This section covers topics not discussed in the other chapters. Some of these things may seem like common sense, but it's the awareness of an issue and providing a remedy that will bring that curl around. So here are some curl bits and tips to help bring out the best curl in you.

Curl Pattern Affected Around Face

Causes: Ponytails, hair ties, pulling hair back when wet

Do you frequently pull your hair back in a tight ponytail and find that the uniform curls you used to have at the sides around your ears are not so curly anymore? Consider it could be the stress you put on those pieces every time you pull your hair back to secure it. You may even find that those two side sections framing your face by your ears, and even the top of your hair, seem to grow longer than anywhere else on your head. Pulling the hair is just like braiding and will, in some cases, increase hair growth—but not in a good, healthy way. (So don't go running to the drugstore to buy every elastic available to tie your hair in a ponytail to increase hair growth!)

The front hairline is the most fragile area of your curly mane, and hair is more fragile when wet than dry. If you pull your hair back in a ponytail when your curls are wet, you will see even more extreme effects on your side pieces: the stress of the elastic pulling on the curls compromises your hair's elasticity and you are actually relaxing your curls and curl pattern in a non-chemical way. And then you likely add on top of that a third curly hair bad habit: using gels and hair spray on wet or dry hair to smooth out those flyaways for a sleek look. Your curls won't only be straighter when you try to go curly, they will be extremely frizzy, too. Alcohol in the gels and hair spray dries out the hair.

This triple threat—tying back *wet* hair and setting with *gel* and *hair spray*— will greatly affect your hairline's curl pattern. Worse than that, if you tug hard enough and/or spray the hairline often enough, your hairline will begin to recede! This means you've damaged the hair that frames your face so much that it will no longer grow there. That, my curl friend, is not a good look for anybody. The best way to secure your hair is loosely with a lace-style elastic pony tie. These will not provide the same support as fabric-covered elastics, but they will put less stress on the hair. Claw-style clips used to secure the front curls back when they are dry are also a solution. Loosely tying back hair, using either method, to avoid stress on the curls at the hairline is important to remember.

> ***Note:*** *There are alcohol-free gels and hair sprays available at salons, beauty supply outlets and some health food stores. You will have to do your research by reading labels. I would opt for a spray bottle or pump hair spray instead of an aerosol, as the butane that assists in pressurizing the spray can also be drying to the curls. Make your own hair spray. Refer to the "Product Knowledge" chapter for the recipe.*

Alcohol-free products may reduce the dryness, but the straightening effect of the pony tie will still compromise the curl pattern. Be gentle with your hair. Don't do anything excessive in any part of your routine. Use moderation as your guide and you will be on the right track.

Improper Conditioning Results in Dry Hair, Predominantly at the Crown Area

Another interesting thing I come across with new clients is complaints of dry curly hair patches on the back portion of their head, the crown area. In most cases, this occurs because you may have applied your conditioner everywhere, as a good curly would, but it's being rinsed out while you shower and turn your back to the water stream. Most conditioners need at least two to three minutes to be effective. The solution is to clip your hair up after putting in the conditioner and cover with a plastic cap. Simple as that.

You're a "Blow-Dry Bangs" Curly or a "Random Curling Iron" Curly

The blow-dryer can affect the elasticity of the hair as much as any other heat appliance, like a flat iron or curling iron. You won't be able to see the full curl potential in your bangs and have them hold their curl pattern until you stop blow-drying and stretching out this area with a brush, as you've been doing. The same goes for the odd little piece you have been curling with an iron. If you want to have the best results for your curls and want the curl to hold, you have to stop compromising the hair's elasticity, which is what you're doing when you use hot tools like curling irons on your bangs. The end result is, when you try to go curly, those areas are more prone to frizz, since you've been dehydrating the curls with these methods. Curl recovery in these cases will depend on the amount of damage done to the curl from the stretching or ironing. Condition these areas well with deep conditioning or light protein treatments once a week; hopefully you have not destroyed the curl pattern past the point of no return, and your curls will bounce back and the frizz will subside as the elasticity is restored.

Otherwise, you will have to wait until your bangs grow out if the damage is too extensive.

"I shed so much when I wash my hair!" — Washing Patterns

So, you're great with your washing routines. You've got your ABCs down. You've reduced the frequency of washing, you're using sulfate-free shampoo and are conditioning properly. But you still find you're shedding a lot. Don't try to stretch your wash days too much or you'll find you will get more tangles and end up pulling out more good, non-shedding hair with the loose ones. Cleansing, co-washing or wet downs every three days may work better than every four or five days. Yes, we naturally lose a certain amount of hair daily. Those with straight hair, in most cases, will not see this loss as much, as the loose hairs blow away in the wind and drop right from the hair as they go about their day. But those of us with curlier hair patterns shed hair directly on our head of curls, which then catch on other curly strands and stay there until wash day. Also know that at certain times of the year, we lose a little more or less hair. Other factors—like medicine, health, pregnancy—affect the shedding, too. Make sure you don't stretch your washing times too much to prevent excessive tangling and shedding.

Identify Different Applications for Different Curly Areas on Your Head

Get to know your hair and curl pattern if you have different patterns in different areas of your head. Use products in different places to provide the style and curl support you need there.

For example:

- Crown frizz requires using leave-in conditioner when applying styling product to wet hair, or sealing with alcohol-free spray gel or hair spray when hair is dry to keep that cuticle down and sealed.

- Curls that lie flat at the top of your head may require a lighter product, such as a spray gel instead of a liquid gel, so as not to weigh that area down; or use a foam or mousse at the top.
- Dry, curly areas need to be spot-moisturized with leave-in conditioner for extra moisture.
- On looser sides, where your curls drop more, use a spray gel or mousse and scrunch those curls well with a microfiber towel when styling to maximize curl encouragement.
- If you want a looser curl, scrunch less when styling and use a heavier product, such as a cream leave-in.
- If you want more curl, scrunch more when styling and use gels to hold the curl pattern, finishing with a mousse or foam for extra curl.
- If the crown (or any area of your head) is prone to excessive dryness or has a tighter, drier curl pattern, you may want to use your conditioning treatment in that area for extra moisture.
- If you have tighter curls at the crown, on the sides or at the nape of your neck, feed your hair more conditioner, particularly a richer, more hydrating product, on the drier areas, leaving more of that conditioner in the hair instead of rinsing it out and applying a leave-in conditioner on those specific areas.

Short Curls at the Back of Your Neck

Trying to avoid the look of the inverted ledge you have happening at the nape of your neck? Sometimes you can have a lot of breakage at the nape when you don't know how to take care of your curls (but now you do!). Instead of cutting all your hair short to match those short pieces, you choose to grow it out. Make sure you condition and hydrate that area well if you feel the curls are not growing there, especially if they tangle a lot and you see breakage.

If you want to create some length when styling those shorter pieces so that your finished style doesn't reveal short hair pushing your outer layer of longer hair up and out, apply a styling product such as a cream or leave-in to this area. This will create a little weight and length, whereas using a gel in this area will encourage curls and cause them to bounce more. Right after you've applied your styling product, gently rake your fingers through those shorter curls and pull them down to elongate.

Longer, Looser Curls at the Nape of Your Neck

To fix this unflattering style, apply a spray gel or lightweight foam or mousse at your nape and scrunch well with a microfiber towel to encourage more curl. Spray gels are lighter weight than liquid ones and can provide more bounce to the curl, as the molecules in a spray product are much smaller and can better penetrate the cuticle for curl encouragement. When you find a curly hair expert who specializes in dry cuts, this look will be a thing of the past.

Tighter Curls at the Crown

As mentioned above, hydrate this dry area well. Apply extra moisturizing products such as a spray or cream leave-in conditioners to the crown. Always make sure the moisture level is optimal and that the cuticles are wide open to receive this extra moisture. Work the product in well with your fingers and pinch down on the strands with your thumb and index finger or use a comb or brush to penetrate the cuticles more effectively. Finish by applying an alcohol-free gel to lock in the moisturizing properties of your leave-in to act as a cocoon for the hair. The gel will buffer the effects of the dry air and heat to better protect those curly dry areas.

Frizzy Hairline

Review your steps to ensure you are cleansing your curls with sulfate-free shampoo and, when conditioning, you are properly coating the hairline. Make sure you are using enough product and applying it thoroughly to your hairline, closing and sealing the cuticles with a moisturizing base or leave-in, if necessary. If you're following everything you've learned in *The*

ABCs and are still experiencing frizzy hairline syndrome, there are a couple of things that could be the cause.

1. Your facial cleansing routine could be the culprit. Facial cleansers and bar soaps leave residue and can be just as harsh as the sulfates in shampoos when left on the hairline. Using a headband when cleaning your face and rinsing the hairline well if it's been touched by the facial cleanser will help reduce frizz. If your hairstyling product has been diluted or removed altogether as a result of your facial cleansing routine, do a quick styling product reapplication to the hairline area. You may even want to consider using sulfate- and/or alcohol-free facial cleansers. You've taken the steps to make healthier choices for your curls by going sulfate-free and choosing better ingredients, so why not try the same for your skin? There are many options available in health food stores. You have to think, if these facial products are stripping and drying to your curls, they can't be great for your face, right?

2. Previous styling methods could be a cause of excessive frizz at the hairline. Your prior use of flat irons or blow-dryers may have been so damaging, it could take a while to see the benefits from changes in your routine. Apply a lightweight leave-in spray conditioner to your hands and rub together to create a light film, then gently graze the product over the hairline, in a motion from the face toward the crown, to provide some extra moisture. Repairing this area can take a month or so, and possibly in extreme cases, your curls have to grow out completely first.

Change-of-Season Curls

What causes frizz? Always remember, frizz indicates hair looking for moisture. I have said it once, twice… many times throughout the book. Moisture can be stripped by routines and products and can be restored by routines and products. Something you are doing or not doing in your routine is contributing to this. Make sure you have enough of a moisturizing primer in your hair as a base during these dry times, whether it's leaving some, most or all of your conditioner on your curls, depending on your curl pattern. The last product left in your hair after cleansing—your conditioner—and the first product you apply for styling will be the most important ones that contribute to the finished style. Learn to recognize what your hair needs as the seasons change.

A dry scalp and uncontrollable frizz mean two things: your hair needs extra moisture and the air you are sleeping and living in does as well. Purchase a humidifier for your bedroom. If it's portable, you can move it from room to room when watching TV or working at your computer, then move it back to your bedroom when you go to sleep at night. Personally, I don't believe the humidifying units that attach to furnaces are truly effective. It's impossible for the moisture to travel through all the ducts and vents to the individual rooms in the house to properly hydrate your skin and, more significantly, your curls.

If hair reacts to the change in season by becoming drier and frizzy, add extra moisture with a leave-in conditioner when applying your styling product on your curly wash-and-style day. Apply to the troublesome dry areas of your curls and finger rake or comb through to help hydrate and force extra moisture into the cuticles to control the dryness and frizz. If you have finer hair, a spray leave-in conditioner will penetrate the cuticles more easily, because the molecules of a liquid are smaller than those of a creamy, thicker leave-in conditioner.

> **Note:** *If you use a rich product with thick consistency but need the versatility of using a lighter product, try diluting a small portion with a little distilled water in a spray bottle for a light mist application. You may find the diluted leave-in will penetrate the cuticles better than the original heavier formulation.*

Use alcohol-free gel in the winter as a final layer to seal in all the benefits of your moisturizing base to protect your hair from the dry, heated air of the furnace and the cold air outside. This also works in the summer to protect from the heat of the sun. The gel provides a barrier and cocoons the hair for extra protection during the periods when curls will appear drier and frizzy. The end result is also better day-after curls if you go a little heavier with the amount of styling products you use during these times. The curls may be a little more "crunchy" and stiff as they dry, but they will soften up over time.

Don't be married to a routine for your curls. Depending on how you wear your hair, you may find you need to switch up the products you use in the summer to something different in the winter, or add another layer of product to the routine to make your staple products work.

Winter Hats, Flannel & Fleece

Stay clear of fleece hats and fuzzy scarves on your neckline if your curls are longer and rest there. It's better to use cotton hats and scarves than these unnatural fibers that will just cause frizz. Or, purchase a microfiber hair toque—or grab the hair tube you read about in "Sleeping Curly"—to wear under your favorite fleece or wool hat; the toque will protect against the ill effects of that material grabbing onto each little cuticle, just causing more frizz. Also stay clear of flannel and microfiber pillowcases: you will wake up super-frizzy when you rest your curls on either one of those materials when you sleep!

> **Note:** *You have seen microfiber mentioned above as a good material for a hair towel or hair tube and a bad material for pillowcases. The ideal kind of microfiber material for a hair toque/tube should be lightweight and thin to protect curls while letting the scalp and curls breathe. Avoid plush, fleece microfiber pillowcases and sheets that have a fluffy texture. It will make hair frizzy, because the curls and cuticles grab onto every plush and fluffy fiber!*

Triangular Shapes

All curlies hate what they refer to as the dreaded "triangle," the shape that can result from the weight and balance of your haircut. Hair that is wavy can triangle out just as much as any other curl pattern, so I can't say this shape happens to just one curl pattern. Below are reasons for this curly shape issue and suggestions on how to fix it.

The dry-cut styling technique can target those areas by what I call "cutting the corners" to create more roundness with a longer-layered cut. This doesn't mean your hair has to be long, it just means the layers themselves are longer and cut a few inches from your base length.

If you are growing out your hair and your curls are resting on your shoulders, sometimes your curls will triangle out because of where the hair is lying, not because of the cut itself. So, if you have mid-length hair and its weight is pulling the hair flatter where it sits on the top of your head and your curls are flaring out at the bottom, creating the triangular look, use one of the clipping methods in Chapter 7, "Styling: Adding Volume with Clips," to create lift at the root and give a rounder shape at the top to balance the bottom.

If it's the weight of the individual strands causing hair to triangle out at the bottom, it can only be targeted by alternating cutting techniques to remove this weight and deal with those heavier areas. When you get a haircut (especially a dry cut), the wide, or triangular, look may show up within a short time after the service if your stylist is not trained in other methods to deal with this imbalance at the ends.

If your hair is cut to one length only, the triangle effect at the bottom is unavoidable. A long-layered haircut will help by removing weight from those flared-out bottom corners. This cut doesn't necessarily mean your hair has to be long to have this technique done. The long-layered haircut, by name, is a technique that adds a layer at the lower length of the hair to remove bulk. Alternatively, a shorter layer blended with layers throughout can provide wonderful lift at the top, so hair doesn't lie so flat, as well as provide a balanced shape throughout.

Knowing this information will help you explain to your curly hair stylist more effectively what you wish to have when your hair is cut and styled.

The Wavy Curly: "They've fallen and can't get up!"

The problem with most wavy curlies (especially those with thick hair) is that after washing and styling their hair, the curls start out great, but gravity pulls them down throughout the day, leaving dropped curls. By getting the right cut to remove weight, and using styling methods such as plopping or curl refreshers, you can add bounce back into your hair. Using the correct styling products to support your style will also get better results. Alcohol-free spray gels applied on freshly styled hair will help to reduce this "curl dropping." The spray gel sets the hair much the same way a hair spray does, but without the drying effects of butane and alcohol. Read "Drying Your Curls: Plopping" as a method to revitalize curls and calm the frizz.

I have a client who uses gel on second-day hair to wake up her beach waves. She puts a small amount in her hand, works section by section, then scrunches with a T-shirt to get the waves to form. Spray gels, foams and mousses are lightweight and great for wavy hair, because you'll get more curl and better hold using these lighter styling products so as to not weigh the waves down.

Swimming, and Chlorine or Saltwater Pools

It's best to wet your curls before getting in the water to swim. Think of your hair as a sponge: it will readily absorb the first liquid it comes in contact with. Although wetting your hair first with water won't stop the chlorine from penetrating, it will definitely slow down the process. You can also try coating wet hair with conditioner and putting on a swim cap. As always, rinse your curls really well after swimming; shampoo or cleanse as needed with sulfate-free shampoo, then condition your hair.

After swimming, you can also try a rinse of one part apple cider vinegar and three parts water. Apply solution, let it sit, then rinse clean. Or use one tablespoon of baking soda and one cup of water. Pour on the hair and allow to sit for a minute. If hair feels slimy, it's working! Rinse clean. For either method (cider vinegar or baking soda), follow with conditioner.

Vacation Tips for the Beach Curly

Just as with the swimming notes above, remember that the most important thing is to start off with wet hair (using tap water) before entering any body of water, and always cleanse and rinse the curls well at the end of the day. If you're a beach curly heading out for the day, wet your hair and apply a nice coat of conditioner. You can even mist some lightweight oil on top of your conditioner to provide an extra buffer against the sun, salt and chlorine. Simply clarify your hair when you return from vacation with baking soda, and shampoo as above.

> ***Note:*** *I always take a small plastic jar of rich conditioner with me to the beach and apply as needed. I rinse out my curls midday at the outdoor shower and apply my conditioner, which acts as a buffer to the sun and heat. This keeps curls healthy and hydrated throughout your beach or pool day and can minimize the salt, chlorine and sun damage. I do this daily when on vacation, and even though my blonde highlights get blonder (they wouldn't get quite as light if I wore my baseball cap more often), my curls are not dried out, frizzy or heat damaged when I return home.*

Hard-Water Curlies

For those living in areas with well water, this provides challenges to your curls, because the mineral deposits can weigh down the hair, affecting your curl pattern and leaving your hair lackluster and flat. Try using cider vinegar rinses after washing your curls. Mix ¼ part cider vinegar with ¾ part distilled water in a spray bottle. Some curly clients I know just leave the mixture in their hair. I would do a final rinse with a bottle of filtered water and then condition the hair.

Day-After Hair for Sport Curlies

I'm a sporty curly, but I don't necessarily wash and style my hair after every workout. My styling routine has me going a little heavier with the amount of styling products I use on my curls the first day of cleansing. Then when I work out, I sometimes only have to use a curly refresher, or spray with conditioner and water, and mist all over my head to pump up my curls. Other times I will quickly (for just a second, so as to not dissolve my styling product) let my hair get wet in the shower to refresh my curls. Anything I can do to stretch a wash day, I do! I sweat when I work out and even wear a hat! But, I find by doing any of the above, I can have a quick shower, fluff up my hair with my hands and am good to go after the gym. I don't feel my scalp is dirty, nor does my scalp smell. I have healthy hair with curls that have good memory—and in time, you'll have the same!

For you sporty curlies, it may be hard to resist washing your hair as you used to following each workout. You'll feel sweaty and smelly and uncomfortable unless you wash your curls. If this describes you and you work out every day, just co-wash your curls (using conditioner as your shampoo). As you co-wash, make sure to create a lot of friction with your finger tips when cleaning your scalp. Understand that it takes time for your scalp's sebaceous glands to get used to creating oil at a normal rate now that you have a sulfate-free cleansing routine. Sulfates, as you have learned, strip moisture from the scalp. In turn, the scalp works extra hard to replace the oils removed in an effort to fight back and replenish itself. Therefore, after cutting out sulfates you may find your scalp excessively greasy for a time, and oils can smell! But in my experience, over time the glands will adapt to the new routine and create oil at a normal rate. Your healthy scalp and curls will thank you for not stripping them anymore, and the smell will be a thing of the past.

> **Note:** *Check your hair, and if it looks good, don't be so quick to run to the shower. We often think that when we are sweaty, it's time for a shower. Well, up until now, you may have also thought that you needed to use a shampoo with sulfates! Just change your mindset, and let the look of your curls dictate your actions.*

Alternative Protective Styles for Curls

There are so many methods available for you to explore on the Internet that don't involve heat damage to change up your style. These online tutorials are great for the health and happiness of your curls, far better than a blow-dry and flat-iron style.

Check out these "protective hairstyles" if you're transitioning or simply looking for a change in your curly style:

- soft or hard roller sets
- hair twists
- hair wrap
- finger coil
- braids
- Bantu knots

Different Curls, Different Stages of Our Lives

Curls change throughout our lives. I can't tell you how many times this happens. Curls get thicker, finer, tighter, looser. Changes happen from birth to pre-teen, from teen to young adult. Our curls sometimes experience a change when we have children and, as we get older and if we get ill. It's unpredictable—just like our curls' personality! Try to live in the here and now and learn to love what you have. Look forward as a curly, and don't be locked in the past. You still have beauty in your curls no matter what texture or pattern your hair has evolved into.

Chapter 16

KISS List

When your curly head starts spinning as you dive into *The ABCs*, don't get overwhelmed; refer to the KISS (Keep It Simple Styling) list below to see how simple the steps are to care for your curls.

1. Always use sulfate-free shampoo. (Shampoo less and co-wash more with conditioner.)
2. Clarify once a month depending on product buildup.
3. Use a good conditioner with botanical ingredients and leave some in as your curl pattern requires, plus weekly treatments as needed.
4. Ensure there's the proper amount of moisture in your hair before applying styling product.
5. Apply appropriate styling products in layers—no product cocktail mixes! Use styling products that are alcohol-free and light on oils, or curl-friendlier styling products with cetyl alcohol or water-soluble oils.

6. Scrunch with a microfiber towel or cotton T-shirt to remove moisture and encourage curl.
7. Use clips or Pik to add volume to your curly style.
8. Choose from the best drying methods: air-dry, diffuse, hooded dryer or plopping.
9. Sleep curly: options include the pineapple, claw clip, mesh bandana, hair tube or plopping (NO SATIN BONNETS).
10. Use a curl refresher to wake up your curls in the morning and always fluff at the root. And away you go!

Closing Notes

I have enjoyed creating *The ABCs*. It's been a long road. Many hours, days, weeks, months and years compiling notes and putting to paper what seems ever so easy to do face to face with clients! Being fortunate enough to be in the position to share the curly knowledge I have and be able to reach curlies of all curl patterns near and far is truly a blessing. Every one of you is special and unique—just like the curls on your heads! Some methods you have read about may seem unorthodox, but when dealing with uniqueness, you have to try things a little differently from the norm to find solutions to the challenges that uniqueness presents. All the methods and routines incorporated in the ABCs are interchangeable. Feel free to try a method that is not categorized for your hair type if it appeals to you. It's what's right for you and your curls!

While in curl recovery, you'll be getting to know your curls. Once you've reached your hair goals, it will be up to you to maintain them. If in time a method or product is no longer working the way it used to, change it up. Don't just fall into a curly rut and keep doing the same thing over and over with the same un-curly results. Step back and see what your curls are telling you! Your curl seeking brought you here, and if you have to return to *The*

ABCs as a refresher to get you back on track, I guarantee that you will learn so much more when you read it the second time around.

Take selfies of your blossoming curls and track your progress on your curl journey in the pages provided at the back of this book. Some curlies take a year or longer to see their true curl potential! Hopefully, *The ABCs* has opened your curly eyes, so you have a better understanding of how you can reach your true curly potential and "Always Be Curly"—and love it!

Your curly stylist,
Adina

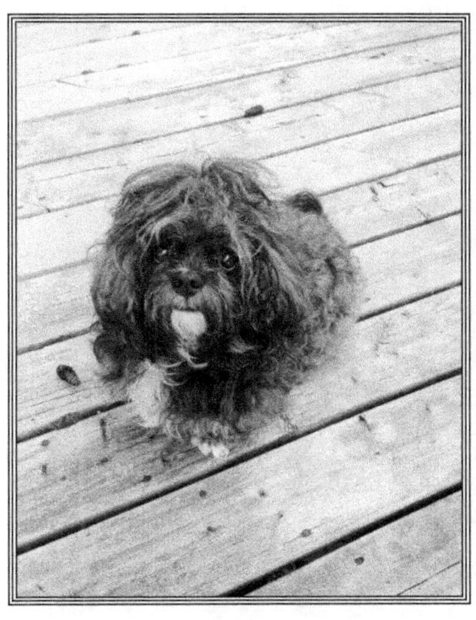

In loving memory of Daisy, my family's sweet Shih-poo who left us in November 2016. She was with me when the studio first opened and stayed with me from the moment I started *The ABCs* until it was completed. A precious little Shih-poo, she curled up beside me for hours, weeks and years while I penned this book. In the studio she touched so many lives with her enthusiastic greetings before excitedly leading clients down the hall to their appointments. Anyone nervous about their first appointment was soon put at ease as Daisy, my curl-therapy pup, distracted them. To me, her unfailing loyalty will be greatly missed but never forgotten. Daisy was truly special.

Life and love are so precious when living yet painful when taken and lost. But I know faith will heal the broken heart—and hope will bring peace.

My Curl Journey Notes...